DIET STARTS
TOMORROW

LOUISE GINGLO

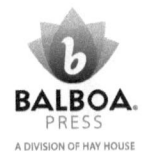

BALBOA.
PRESS

A DIVISION OF HAY HOUSE

Balboa Press books may be ordered through booksellers or by contacting:

Balboa Press
A Division of Hay House
1663 Liberty Drive
Bloomington, IN 47403
www.balboapress.com.au
1-(877) 407-4847

ISBN: 978-1-4525-0954-9 (sc)
ISBN: 978-1-4525-0955-6 (e)

Because of the dynamic nature of the Internet, any web addresses or links contained in this book may have changed since publication and may no longer be valid. The views expressed in this work are solely those of the author and do not necessarily reflect the views of the publisher, and the publisher hereby disclaims any responsibility for them.

The information, ideas, and suggestions in this book are not intended as a substitute for professional medical advice. Before following any suggestions contained in this book, you should consult your personal physician. Neither the author nor the publisher shall be liable or responsible for any loss or damage allegedly arising as a consequence of your use or application of any information or suggestions in this book.

Any people depicted in stock imagery provided by Thinkstock are models, and such images are being used for illustrative purposes only.
Certain stock imagery © Thinkstock.

Printed in the United States of America

Balboa Press rev. date: 03/14/2013

Love yourself first and everything else falls into place. You really have to love yourself to get anything done in this world.

—Lucille Ball

Contents

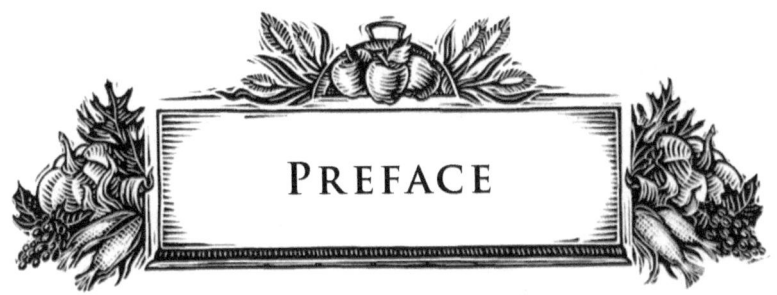

PREFACE

Motivation, inspiration, and recognizing that most of us can relate to each other when it comes to challenges regarding our body image, is what led me to write this book.

From 1998 to the beginning of 2005, I was employed as a Weight Loss Consultant for a major weight loss chain. Moving on from there I had a similar role in a gym. During this time, I consulted many people who struggled with their weight, jumping from one program to another eagerly waiting to see which one would magically work for them. For some clients, the plans I consulted them on, did work—but for others, the ongoing cycle of trying to lose weight continued.

I struggled for many years with my weight, even during my role as a Weight Loss Consultant. From my teen years of being over-weight to my twenty's, where my weight went down, then back up, down a little and up quite a bit again. Finally in my early thirty's I had it all figured out, and have not looked back since.

I discovered how to get healthy and lose weight, on my own. I achieved this by following a healthy balanced eating plan. I never saw it as a diet, and I never told myself or anyone else for that matter, that I was on a diet. I just simply decided it was time to take unhealthy foods, and large meals out of the equation, and got myself moving. I didn't eliminate a food group such as carbohydrates, dairy, or fats (although I am a vegetarian, so technically there was no meat, but I made sure I had plenty of protein).

I also decided that I should never be deprived, or restricted by my healthy lifestyle. I love chocolate, therefore I always made sure I could include it—not every day, but it was definitely a part of my diet a few times a week. My average day consisted of cereal, sandwiches, soups, pasta, legumes, cheese, rice, dairy food, sometimes a little bit of ice-cream, treats here and there, and most importantly a lot of fruit and vegetables.

I cut down on my portion sizes, because really, I was eating like a man. The pasta on my plate exceeded way over what my husband would eat. I used to feel so lethargic and heavy after dinner, and the reason why became obvious to me, once I stopped loading my plate up. It became apparent to me that although I believed I ate healthy foods most of the time, my body was not on a healthy path and it showed in many different ways. I knew too well, that if I didn't take control of this, the result would be me continuing to put on more weight, as well as putting my health at risk.

People began to notice my transformation and were asking me how I was achieving my weight loss. When I informed them of how completing a food journal was part of the healthy lifestyle process, the response from the vast majority was, "Oh, I am too busy for that." I felt like they were implying I had all the time in the world to write out my food for the day. Seriously, it only takes a few minutes to jot down what you just ate, it isn't really that time consuming at all. A journal is a wonderful tool as an in-your-face look at your eating habits, and something to learn from, as well as somewhere to write down feelings, challenges, emotions, and all that comes with any change that shifts your habits and rituals. And most of all, it is MOTIVATING. So, taking the time out to use a journal will become an integral part of an individual's healthy lifestyle journey.

I have become passionate too about people going on what I believe are the wrong weight loss programs. I have seen many people try various diets, or going with the latest fads. There is the detox diet, no carb & low carb diet, soup or liquid diet, no fat, low fat, meal replacement shakes and bars, sugar free, dairy free, and even fruit free (because apparently fructose makes you fat). People are always excited about starting these diets, and they always mentioned how they lost so much in the first week etc, but then I see them a month later, and they are off the diet, and never got to the goal they had in mind when they started.

I find it interesting that not many people become as excited about "eating healthy", as they do about these so called diets. Maybe it is because eating a balanced healthy diet every day doesn't result in you losing a massive amount of weight super fast. This is why we need to change the way we think in terms of dieting and weight loss.

A friend of mine decided she would embark on a weight loss program that consisted of her eliminating foods such as tomatoes, mushrooms, lettuce as well as various other foods that are healthy for our bodies. This plan also didn't allow any snacks in-between her meals. Part of the program was that the dieters had to wait five hours between meals. For example, breakfast, followed by five hours of no food, then lunch, another five hours of no food, then dinner, and then nothing until breakfast the next day. Where would your energy come from to do any exercise, or anything else for that matter?

My friend did lose weight, and she did look good, but the last time I saw her, she had put all that weight back on. My point is, I don't believe there is much to learn, from a program like that. Once the client finishes the program, they are back out there on their own and without learning about their body and what it takes to be healthy, the right way.

To be honest I have never seen anyone actually succeed long-term on any of those diets, and yes I have been guilty of giving them a go myself, without success. They will work for while because quite frankly any diet where you take away a whole group of food, will work if you focus on it and are strict with yourself. But what do you learn from it? You learn that in order to lose weight, you have to deprive yourself of things you love, as well as following a menu plan that is unrealistic and inconvenient, and even more so, when you try to socialize.

Since I started my healthy lifestyle, about ten years ago, I have maintained my weight (I did lose more a couple of years ago, by going even healthier), and I have adopted a different way of thinking, when it comes to food. Although I still have sugar in my diet, it doesn't come in the form of cakes, cookies, ice-cream and desserts. If I do feel the urge to consume one of the previous listed items, I go to buy it, but then all I can see is SUGAR. I have created a click in my mind that tells me to stop before I buy, even though somewhere else in my mind I really wanted that piece of junk. There are occasions where I will have a treat, but I try to save it for birthdays, holidays, a day out with friends, or a special event. Therefore, I could go weeks without having any cake or months without ice-cream. This is just one example, but I do it with many foods, especially take-away which I hardly eat.

Most of the time people are so focused on just losing the weight, and wanting a quick fix, they are forgetting about eating a balanced diet that includes all five food groups, and improving their health. It's time to say "no" to dieting, and "yes" to "I want to be healthy now, and for the rest of my life."

I want people to be motivated to reach for the stars when it comes to their health. If the focus becomes your health, and reaping the rewards of maintaining a healthy body, then there should be no more failure, because you will stop feeling deprived, punished and restricted. It's time to live life to the fullest, with a healthy body and mind.

INTRODUCTION

I have always loved reading success stories where others have pursued a healthy lifestyle that also led them to reducing their weight. I found these to be motivating, moving and inspiring. I always wanted the stories to go further and have me being able to dig deeper into the minds of these individuals who became successful in beginning, and then maintaining a healthy lifestyle.

Although Ruby is a fictional character, her story is very real. Follow her journey of how she feels about her weight, her body, how she thinks others view her and, her many dieting failures, and then find yourself inspired by her transition into a new woman both inside and out.

This book does not set out a menu plan for you to follow, nor does it have recipes of healthy foods to eat. The aim of this story is to help you get motivated, and start on your own healthy lifestyle. You could choose a program out there to suit you and your everyday needs and use this book to motivate you along the way. Or you could decide to follow your own healthy path and use this book as your companion for daily inspiration while on your path to success.

CHAPTER 1

Diet starts tomorrow . . . . again. This is what I tell myself when I have ruined a day that was meant to be the start of yet another diet.

I began my diet this morning and all was good, that is until I went to work. A slice of cake was shoved in front of my face and they told me I would lose my job if I didn't have a piece. Well, that is how is went down in my mind.

I wouldn't have started my diet today if I knew it was Sheree's birthday. Seriously, it seems like every second day at the office, it is someone's birthday—I wish I had been fired. I need a new job where people don't have any birthdays.

So it was only one piece of cake, I hear all the professional dieters out there saying "just get back up again! Don't let one failing be the ruler of your whole day." True, I must admit, I could have gone and bought a bunch of lettuce from the supermarket, eaten that for my lunch, and then taken a walk around the city for 45 minutes. I would now be praising myself for eating like a rabbit and getting in some exercise, but I didn't. Who starts a diet on a Friday anyway?

I am really disappointed in myself. I have wasted a day of losing weight. Today could have been worth 500 grams down on the scales. Who am I kidding? Maybe I am just meant to be this way, maybe, I am supposed to be 100 kilos for the rest of my life! I am not meant to be skinny! This is what I tell myself every time I slip up, and ruin my diet. It is a vicious circle of mind talk and self punishment and ultimately

1

why I fail. And then at the end of the day I go home and eat a huge bowl of pasta big enough to feed an entire Italian family.

I have always been overweight. Even as a child I was always told I was fat. I was teased constantly, not only by the boys from the Catholic School up the road, who made elephant gestures at me as I walked past them but also from young family members, such as cousins. I have acknowledged over the years that being fat, is who I am and maybe that is the way I am meant to stay.

I remember when I was about ten, my aunt (who is only two years older than me) held up a tennis racket, turned it sideways and told me that the round part of the racket was my butt and the handle part was my thighs. Now, she wasn't saying my thighs were as thin as the handle but she was remarking to me that my butt stuck out . . . . a lot, just like the racket. I can laugh at it now, because I think it is quite a funny analogy—my big round behind, sticking out, bulging like a racket, who would have thought?

High School was just as bad, if not worse, as you can imagine, the boys were always telling me how fat and ugly I was and come to think of it the girls were pretty good at it too. Not to mention the fact that my parents thought it would be great to name me Ruby. Oh people love the name NOW. It wasn't lovely when I was a child and far from being popular like it is today. Now, lots of cute little baby girls are given that name and it is in the top 20 list of popular names! Not when I was born though. Names like Michelle, Sarah, Melissa and Jessica were the way to go, not RUBY!

I found some friends that were like me, slightly overweight, freckly, bad hair, and just plain awkward looking and even though we may not have had a lot in common in our likes and dislikes, we made it work because quite frankly we had no one else. Even the geeky guys didn't like us because fantasy took over and they all kept thinking that one day soon, they would get one of the pretty girls from the cool or prissy cliques.

So, here I am today at age 26 still struggling with my oversized curves and the rolls that protrude from every part of my body, determined each day that 'this is the day' I will conquer my fat demons. I am not complaining or feeling sorry for myself, I know I am mostly to blame. My family aren't big like me, my parents are a normal weight and my mother fed us a healthy diet—maybe she was too strict, I could blame it on that couldn't I?

My sister Emerald (yes Emerald, but at least she could shorten it and fool people, "just call me Emmy" she would say) is a perfect size 8 of course. Emmy is cute, pretty and petite. She is lovely too and one of my biggest supporters. She is younger than me, twenty four and she just got married. I was shocked when she asked me to be her Maid of Honour because I really didn't believe she would want me to be part of the bridal party. I did look out of place, all of Emmy's friends are slim like her and looked so beautiful in their strapless bridesmaid dresses fitted to the waist and then slightly flowing out over their lovely cute round button butts. Being the Maid of Honour we were able to get away with a different style of dress to suit my "over emphasized body parts" as the lady in the bridal store put it. I think she was trying to be polite but it really didn't work.

I had a year before the wedding to get myself in order, but not even that was enough motivation for me to slim myself into a beautiful gown. I tried, I really did try but obviously not hard enough and I do regret it. The one time I have been asked to be a bridesmaid and I looked liked a whale in a lilac dress.

You see, I am the very well maintained fat lady. I never find it difficult to get a job. I often receive compliments about my clothes, hair, make-up, shoes, handbags and nails. It's nice to get compliments, but instead of being told I look great or pretty in something, I get comments such as "I like your dress" or "Love the shoes Ruby." So really the compliments are about the things I choose, not on how I look in those things. I like to keep myself well dressed. I spend money on all the things I need to keep myself looking as classy as I possibly can.

As a paralegal and personal assistant for a lawyer in a major city firm, I earn really good money. I live on my own in a nice townhouse near the beach and I now have great women friends who love and support me.

Of course, there are things missing. I would like a loving partner and to have children. I have had a couple of boyfriends, one serious relationship (with a guy named Jake) when I was about 23 years old. It lasted for 12 months and we broke up. I am still not completely sure why, I think he loved me but his friends didn't. He didn't seem to mind my weight. He always told me I was beautiful but I know his friends made fun of me and they all had thin girlfriends, I never felt like I fit in with them. It's sad but true that we are all judged by the way we look and it's worse when we are young especially in the twenty's age group, the time of going out, looking sexy and being able to wear fantastic little black dresses with plunging necklines, or little shorts on the weekends and summer dresses.

Yep, no more excuses, but this time the journey is for me and no one else. I need to feel good and know that I am healthy. I have to stop dieting with the aim of looking good, or to fit into a pair of size 12 jeans, or to wear a nice dress to a wedding. Hell, I have nice, in fact I have beautiful dresses in my closet already . . . . this will now be about my health and nothing else!

There's one hour to go before work finishes and my phone rings "Hey Ruby!" My friend Michelle is on the other end, "want to join me for some dinner tonight? I was thinking I might invite myself over to your place and we can make something yummy—low joule of course." "Sounds great to me, see you at 6.30?" "Excellent, see you then."

I love Michelle she is one of my best friends. We met at college when we were both nineteen. She also works as a paralegal for another firm in the city. Michelle is bright, fun and attractive. She is not afraid to say what she thinks and she always makes people laugh. She is thin but never makes me feel uncomfortable about the way I am. She doesn't have a boyfriend at the moment but is never short of admirers and I love hearing her stories about the many dates she goes on with the strange guys she seems to attract. Usually when we get together, we talk about my constant mission for thinness and her adventures at finding a long term boyfriend.

It's finally time to finish up work for another week and I decide to go get a few things from the supermarket before heading home. I pick up some chips, crackers, dip, cheese, frozen pizza and of course dessert—I go with the cheesecake. Oh and I can't forget to pop into the bottle shop for a couple of bottles of red wine.

I get home and Michelle is there within half an hour. It doesn't take us long to get stuck into the wine and nibbles. I love doing this! Sitting with one of my best friends having a good old chat and eating, munching, drinking and more eating, I mean is there anything better? But of course a little over half way through the night, and one bottle of wine later, I am feeling guilty yet again and I start to have a melt down over all the food sins I have committed in just one night.

"Please don't get mad at me" Michelle starts to say, "but I had another reason for coming over tonight, other than pigging out. A lady I work with has lost a substantial amount of weight, looks super healthy and happy, so I asked her how she did it. She told me she did it through a Healthy Lifestyle Coach. Apparently she has a different way of approaching weight loss or it isn't actually about weight loss, it was a bit confusing. Anyway Rhonda, (the lady from work) says she loved going for her sessions with this coach."

"I'm not mad" I say to her, "in fact I was thinking about losing weight again today, after I failed miserably on the diet I started this morning (as usual), but this time I promised myself it would be about being healthy and not about reaching a certain number on the scale by Christmas or to fit into an amazing dress etc. So, did you get her name and number for me?"

"Of course!" she says excitedly. And I vow to my dear friend that I will be making the call first thing in the morning, and after hearing a little more about this Healthy Lifestyle Coach—Crystal, (she even has a skinny person's name), I am feeling slightly excited.

CHAPTER 2

Nine o'clock on the dot, I ring the phone number and of course I get a message asking me to leave my name and number, which I do. While I am sitting waiting for the call that is going to change my life I find myself wondering whether I should start eating healthy today or if I should just continue with my normal Saturday routine. That is, buy a magazine from the newsagent, sit in my favourite café which also happens to be the best patisserie, order a coffee and have something yummy from their vast selection of indulgent cakes, slices and tortes. Hmm, what to do? What to do? The phone rings. Well I think fate has made the decision for me.

It is Crystal and I am glad. She informs me that she keeps her Saturday's free for any new clients, as well as existing clients that need that little bit of extra help, or motivation for the weekend. I am booked in to see her at 1pm which is perfect because now I have to behave otherwise I am sure she will sense the guilt I will be feeling if I am slacking off today.

I arrive at her office. It's at the back of a new age shop which is different, but I love it. I walk into the waiting area. There are a couple of wind chimes hanging from the ceiling and they gently blow in the breeze that is flowing in through the open door. I can hear the trickling of water running through a small water fountain that sits on a side table. There is a two seater lounge along one side of the room and a three seater down the other side. Usually I have to plant my big butt on uncomfortable plastic chairs in all the other waiting rooms I have ventured into. On the walls, hang a couple of those inspirational posters that have beautiful, serene pictures. It is pretty much like the shop out the front—welcoming and relaxing. I pick a spot on one of the sofas and I wait.

Within five minutes Crystal walks out of the office and into the waiting room. She is saying good bye to another client. A woman that looks fresh and healthy or maybe I just think she does, because she is here . . . . nope, she does. She even gives Crystal a big hug before she walks out the door and gives me a big smile. The smile tells me she knows my reason for the appointment and it is meant to reassure me that I am in the right place.

Crystal gestures for me to enter her office which is pretty much like the waiting room, it is relaxing and comfortable very unlike other offices I have visited when enquiring about getting rid of my over-sized body. Most often they are very clinical and hard on the eyes, making it impossible to concentrate with the fluorescent lights, white walls and stark surroundings.

Crystal is of average height and lean (of course), but healthy lean. She doesn't have the too skinny I can eat anything look. She is brunette with gold highlights and has an attractive friendly face, she is older than me, maybe by about ten years and I instantly feel comfortable sitting across from her. She doesn't have a big desk in the middle of the room to navigate our meeting but instead uses a coffee table with one single seater lounge chair at one end and another one to the side. It is a nice arrangement almost as if I were sitting having coffee with a friend.

Crystal has asked me to fill in some forms. There are the usual medical background questions, as well as noting any previous diets I have been on before. Where do I start? I am not sure if the space given is big enough for the list of programs I have tried. From the time I was fourteen, I have tried diets where meals are provided, food is counted, calories added up, fads where I eat nothing but soup for five days, no carbs, low carbs, no fat, no sugar, flush out your system toxin freeing diets, etc, etc. I have also had many visits to weight loss consultants, gyms, nutritionists, and dietitians. Hmmm, maybe I will just write "all of them" in the space—that basically says it all.

After perusing my information, Crystal starts by asking me what my goals are, and my thoughts on how I hope she can help me.

"Ah, ultimately I would like to lose 40 kilos and I am hoping you can help me achieve that by whipping me out of being a total pig" I say, hoping to add a little bit of humour. I fail miserably. She doesn't laugh (at all) but says with a gentle smile on her face "Ruby, what you want to achieve will never happen if you keep referring to yourself as a pig, or any other labels relating to being a pig, fat, over-sized etc. You are a beautiful human being who needs some guidance in changing your lifestyle. So, no more negative talk about yourself, okay."

I stare at her stunned. She wasn't rude or stern, she was compassionate and caring. No one in my life has ever told me, not talk about myself in that way. Yes, they all do the "oh, Ruby you're not a pig" or "you're not fat" and wave their hands as if to get rid of my comments into the thin air but never literally made me realize how wrong this self talk was.

Tears start welling and she looks at me with concern in her eyes, "you know, it's bad enough when other people talk about you, tease you, be rude about your weight, or make rude gestures toward you regarding your body size but you are the only person you can count on to be kind to you. It is normal to put up a shield in order to protect yourself and in doing that, it is common to use humour to try and lighten the subject of your weight. But in doing so, you are telling yourself and the universe it is ok for you to be disrespected and treated unkindly, making these comments or jokes about yourself, gives everyone else permission to behave this way toward you too.

Wow! Floored me once again, and I have a light bulb moment. Crystal has made me aware that I always make jokes or call myself fat names because I am constantly worried that someone else is going to do this, so I try and beat them to it.

Before I can reflect too long on this she quickly changes the subject, in order get the session moving on I guess. Anyway, I have plenty of time at a later stage to sit and think about what I have just learned about myself.

"You mentioned you wanted to lose 40 kilos, where did that number come from?" She says. "Well", I say a little embarrassed "I think I am about a hundred kilos and well sixty kilos is that magic number." I cringe wondering if she thinks that is an impossible goal for me to reach.

"Okay. And how do you want to get to that number" she says, and I am surprised but at the same time I know she has more to say on that but not at this moment. "Well, I want to go on a diet. But I want to be healthy. In general, I already am healthy. I have no major health concerns and my blood pressure and cholesterol are fine—but for how long? Plus, I am aware that I am not as healthy as I could be. I want to learn how to be healthy and stay healthy. It's not like I eat junk food every day or I don't know what a salad is, or what good food is even, I just don't know how to make it work for me. And I'll be honest in saying that yes, I do like bad food and I probably have a little too much of it." Phew, there, I got it all out.

Her face softens once again as if she is about to tell me about some secret magic potion she has gotten a hold of—no . . . . wait, that would be too easy. "I am sure you noticed I am called a Healthy Lifestyle Coach" she says smiling. I nod. "I don't use the word diet because as you just told me, you want to become healthy and stay that way which means you want it to be part of your lifestyle, forever. So I am glad to hear you want to be healthy, because it is the first step in becoming aware this isn't just about being on a program for ten weeks, six months or a year, this is about changing your life for the better and keeping it that way".

"That's where Healthy Lifestyle comes into my title, and Coach is because I am here to train and guide you. The way you think about food and your body is going to change. I am here to guide you, not to tell you what to do. I am also going to help you become in—tune with your body, what it needs and eventually being able to recognize what it doesn't need and how it feels when you have gone too far. You might also find it interesting to know, that not all of my clients are overweight. I also have quite a number of people that come to me who are thin, but realize they aren't as healthy as they could be—so, they come to me to get motivated and advice on how to lead a new healthy lifestyle."

Wow—it had never occurred to me that a person who I would consider to be lean and healthy would need guidance on how to eat well. It does make sense. I mean I have friends that are thin but don't necessarily eat any better than I do, maybe just smaller portions of what I would eat, maybe they skip meals to stay thin, and some of them are more active than what I am.

I am starting to feel excited, Crystal is motivating me already and we haven't even touched the surface of where I am heading.

"One of the most important things you will be doing for yourself is a daily journal. This isn't just to record what you eat for the day as well as any activity you do but I also want you to write down any thoughts you have—negative or positive. Any experiences and challenges you encounter through people, events, something at work or while shopping. Anything that puts you on a high or sends you spiraling down, whatever you feel the need to write, you write it. The diary is for you, I won't be reading it when you come in for a session, but I am happy to discuss anything you are proud of yourself for, as well as anything that upset you or you found challenging."

I am looking at her and before I have a chance to burst into song about how busy I am as a Paralegal and P.A, she continues with "and I don't want to hear about how too busy you are to write in a journal. If you have time to go home after work and decide you don't feel like cooking and then go get take-away, you have time for a journal. If you have a craving for something sweet and you take a trip to the supermarket to buy it, then you have time for a journal." That is so true, I feel like I am sinking into the chair out of embarrassment for even considering the 'I'm too busy speech'.

We are already half-an-hour in and she hasn't mentioned food yet. "So what um menu plan do I follow" I say carefully avoiding the word 'diet'.

"Good question" she says laughing a little for the first time. She then gives me a quick rundown of what living a healthy lifestyle consists of for example salad with my meals, lean meats, a breakfast that doesn't consist of ten teaspoons of sugar, and options for healthy snacks. Most of this I already know from my previous adventures into this well-known world of dieting but it is always good to have a brief refresher course.

"We won't be setting up a menu plan for you to follow" she says. "Okay" I say with hesitance and feeling a little confused. Now I am wondering if this is the right way to go for me, I mean I feel like I need someone to tell me what to do and which direction to head in. Almost as if she has read my mind, she continues "For the first week, I want you to eat what you think is needed for a healthy lifestyle change. And I need you to write down what you eat so I can read it when you come in next week and we can go through it together. Keep this separate to your private journal."

"What if I do something wrong" I say with concern to her. "There is no such thing as wrong Ruby. Remember, you are not on a diet, just be mindful of what you are about to put into your body, and you will know what is right. Believe in yourself. You have made the first step, now you just have to put on your new shoes and walk the path."

Hmm . . . . I like that—Ruby's new shoes. I am ridding myself of the comfortable baggy shoes I put on every day, and replacing them with the new ones which will be uncomfortable to begin with but I will eventually get used to them and walk with new pride and comfort.

"So remember to bring your food journal for me to see next week as it will give me an opportunity to see what you like to eat and if there is something in there that isn't the best option I can help by giving you an alternative to that particular choice. I don't believe in depriving ourselves of the things we enjoy. There is always a way to fit in the things we like. I also believe moderation and portion size is the key when it comes to eating and you will see what I mean by this when I give you your kit to take home."

Ah, a kit, now I am feeling slightly better. The kit must have hints, ideas, recipes something to help me out.

"Another thing I want to touch on before you go," she says. "I think 40 kilos is a lot to aim for in the beginning. I mean does that number overwhelm you?"

"Yes!" I say a bit louder than I planned. "It completely overwhelms me. That is three quarters the weight of one of my friends. It sounds unreachable and like it would take me ten years to get to."

"Well embarking on a healthy lifestyle means there are no numbers, I don't want you thinking of a number. There is no more sixty. It is now just about making better choices and feeling good about them. You need to be kind to yourself and giving yourself this huge pressure to reach a certain number on a scale is not going to help."

I do agree and I believe it has been a huge barrier for me every time I try to lose weight. It sits over my head like a big sign and then it sits on my head, then my shoulders and weighs me down even more than the actual weight I have on my body.

"Also, tell me something you like about yourself" she says, scanning me. I think for moment without saying a word. Does she mean internally or externally? I am not sure, so I mutter "um I am a hard worker." How lame was that? I sounded like a school girl going for her first job interview.

"I am happy and not surprised to hear that Ruby, I am sure you are" Crystal says, trying hard to get me over my embarrassment. "How about something else" she says, prompting me that it wasn't quite the answer she was looking for.

"Um . . . ." this is hard, but why? "I have good taste in clothes." I think Crystal realizes that at this point I am a lost cause for trying to find something nice to say about myself and she lets me off the hook.

"Well next week when you come in, I want you to be able to tell me three things you like about yourself. I don't want it to be all about your personality either. Find some external things too, for example, I have pretty eyes. I am kind or I treat my body well by putting nutritional foods into it. These are all perfect examples of finding things that you like about yourself. Eventually I will hear you replace the word 'like' with 'love'."

So the approach is: no diet, no number for the scales, must do food diary, must do personal journal for me, find things I like about myself, no negative self talk or bad jokes and I need to enjoy myself and give praise for the change I am about to embark on.

Before I leave, Crystal weighs me but I am not allowed to look at the scale. She advises me that her jotting down the number is purely for her records but I can see them much later down the track if I choose to. Crystal also measures my bust, waist, arms, hips and thighs and although I have had this done so many times before, I am still not over the embarrassment of having a tape measure stretched around me to result in large numbers scrawled onto a piece of paper. Plus I always worry that the tape won't actually reach the whole circumference of me—does it then revert back to zero if this happens? I choose not to look at my measurements, even though I was given the option.

I am given my kit and we go through it together. "So in here there are a couple of health magazines for women. I find they are motivational and have lots of good articles and advice in them. There are some handouts I have printed up myself which include meal ideas, what to snack on, how to include activity into your day, some affirmations and visualization tools to help you get through the day, and a brand new bowl and plate."

What? I have never been given a brand new bowl and plate on any program before, food maybe, but not bowls, or plates. And they are the size you would give to a small child . . . . I don't get it. I must have been looking at her like she had four heads so she goes on to explain that these are for me to use so I get used to smaller portion sizes. Oh! Now I get it. A small bowl so I don't load up the cereal, pasta, or rice and a small plate so I don't overfill it for dinner etc. If it's too big for the dish, then it's too big for my stomach. "Feel free to weigh or measure anything" she said, "but this is an easier way to do it."

My hour is up and I leave feeling good. I realize I have a bit of reading ahead of me and I am tempted to get myself some "perusal items" (that means coffee and cake or chocolate biscuits). I stop myself as I am sure that it is not what I am meant to do after spending an hour with my Healthy Lifestyle Coach.

CHAPTER 3

I arrive home and before settling down to look through my kit, I do decide to go with a coffee, surely I am able to include that into my new lifestyle.

I flick through the magazines just to get an idea of what is in them and I am feeling motivated already. I will be able to spend tomorrow reading through them more thoroughly. I come across the handouts and I already like some of the meal suggestions and so I stick these on my notice board in the kitchen for easy referencing.

I am also loving the mini booklet that includes success stories from previous clients, ideas for getting activity into my day (walking up the stairs at work instead of using the lift) yes, I can use that one for sure. The affirmations are very inspiring, such as 'I am a healthy beautiful person' 'I will only put foods that are beneficial to me in my body' 'I am not fat, I am healthy' and so on. I place those on the notice board as well so I can read them daily.

What I really love is the advice given for when times get tough. For example, if I have a sugar craving, I need to stop before reaching for anything sweet and ask myself why I want this. Is it because I am hungry? If the answer is 'no', then I am probably wanting it just for something to do and to get that quick sense of gratification, which means I shouldn't reach for the sugar. If the answer is 'yes, I am hungry' then why am I wanting something that has no nutritional value to it and will not be beneficial to my body or health and will only lead to me wanting something else within half an hour.

These are things I have always known. I mean I am not completely oblivious to the fact that food such as vegetables, fruits, dairy, good oils and lean meats have important vitamins and minerals that contribute to us being healthy, it just never dawned on me to adopt this way of thinking when beginning a diet before. I mostly took a shallow approach and just bought the program that was required walked away and tried to stick to it. I would then battle with my mind knowing I was "dieting" and then start resenting the fact that I had to diet, while other people around me didn't. The fact that I could never just enjoy myself with food depressed me. Why can't I be that skinny girl sitting at the table across from me in the food court eating a fattening take away without feeling so guilty?

I later wrote all of that down in my journal.

I have become so engrossed with my reading material I have forgotten all about having a snack. My stomach starts to rumble so I decide I should see what options I have in the kitchen. I always buy fruit, so I go with an apple. I remembered I had some nuts in the pantry, so I also eat a handful of almonds as well as some cranberries. It was actually a satisfying quick bite and I feel better than I would have if I were to have sat down with a sweet treat.

My phone rings and I have a feeling before I even look at it that it is Michelle checking to see how I went at my appointment. I am right. "Hi, how has your day been?" I dive straight into asking her a question because I know she is dying to ask me a question first. "Good" she says, "relaxing. How was your session with Crystal?" "Great!" I say enthusiastically, "much better than I was expecting. I love her. I think she is actually going to be able to help me." The rest of our conversation is me filling Michelle in about what Crystal is like and how she works with clients and guides them on their journey. She can tell I am excited and she genuinely sounds happy for me.

"Do you feel up to going out tonight?" she asks. "Sam, Danni and Nat want to go out too." "Sounds great! I'm starting a healthy lifestyle, it's not like I've just been diagnosed with something horrible" I say to her with a little chuckle. Before hanging up, I offer to drive so that I am not tempted to drink more than what I think I should. I pat myself on the back for actually following one of the suggestions in the booklet on coping with going out.

Before getting ready to go, I look up the restaurant on the internet and check out their menu (another hint from the book), this allows me to see what is available and I can have the meal I want to choose set in my mind, that way I am less likely to change it. I am thankful they have an oven prepared fish meal with steamed vegetables and I am looking forward to it. I also check out the dessert menu because I know all the other girls will have something after dinner and I thought I should brace myself for being disappointed now rather than later. There is ice-cream served with fruit salad and I decide I can go with that if I feel the need to. I am now feeling much better about going out and I am excited that it can be done. Healthy Lifestyle, here I come!

Saturday August 4th, 11.30pm

Dear HJ (healthy journal),

Tonight I went out with friends to a restaurant. It is the first night of my journey to become a healthier me. I am glad I drove which meant I only had one glass of wine. For the rest of the night, I drank water. I ordered fish and vegetables for dinner and I was grateful they didn't seem to be too oily. I am also proud of myself for asking that the creamy sauce be put on the side, which I didn't touch at all.

Things were going well and I was enjoying just being out with friends and having great conversation. When it came time to order dessert, I decided I wasn't that hungry after all and I would stick with just a coffee. One of my friends (Danni) started pushing me to have dessert "oh come on, you only live once. It's only for tonight" I kept hearing her say these things over and over . . . . it was really getting to me. Danni is the only one of my friends that it also overweight. I think she was trying to sabotage me. All the other girls were telling her to quit and she finally listened—thank god. So, I just ordered a coffee, which came with a small dark chocolate, which I ate. I am feeling fine about eating that little bit of chocolate, because I am not on a diet, I am simply changing to make healthier choices.

I felt good about what I ate at the restaurant and I know I can look forward to going out with friends again.

They all wanted to go dancing afterwards but I am not into being at nightclubs at this stage of my life and although it would have been a great way to get in some natural activity, I decided to go home. Plus an early night means I am more likely to get up in the morning and go for a walk along the beach.

Goodnight, feeling good Ruby.

Sunday August 5th 9.45pm

Dear HJ,

I wasn't sure what to have for breakfast, so I had fruit salad and a tablespoon of yogurt. Then I went for a walk down to the beach and strolled along the sand—I was gone for 1 hour. It wasn't a power walk and I didn't sweat or feel like I had run a marathon, but I feel even a stroll at this point is a great start. I haven't done any exercise for a long time so I feel the need to start slow.

When I came home, I took my time having a shower. After getting dressed, I made a coffee put some clothes in the washing machine and sat down to read the newspaper while drinking my coffee.

I was getting hungry so I ate a handful of almonds and about eight rice crackers. As I didn't get a chance to do any housework yesterday, I thought it was a good idea to do some today and it was a great way to keep myself occupied until lunchtime.

For lunch I usually have a toasted cheese sandwich. You know the kind where you butter both sides of the bread, place the cheese in the middle and then put them in a hot pan, the cheese is all yummy and gooey and melted, and the bread is oily. Well I usually have two sandwiches but today I didn't. Instead, I had ham, lettuce and tomato on two slices of bread with grated carrot, chopped celery, a little bit of grated cheese with sultanas on the side. By the time I finished I felt comfortable, I knew I hadn't eaten too much and it was yummy.

I spent the afternoon looking through the magazines Crystal provided me with and I read some helpful and interesting articles. I also planned my week going through what food choices will be best while I am at work. I am now feeling confident that I can make it happen while at the office.

Dinner was homemade vegetable soup with half a cup of pasta thrown into it. After dinner I ate a small frozen yogurt, I am not sure if this is the right choice, but I felt as though I needed something just to fill that void.

All in all I feel good, I know it is only the first full day but it feels different to any other time and I think it is because I feel like I am in charge of my diet and not someone else. I am the one that gets to make the choices so it makes me stop and think about what I need rather than what I have to have because it is written on a menu plan or it is sitting in my fridge waiting for me.

Good night journal ☺

Monday August 6th 8.30pm

Dear HJ,

Before getting out of bed, I took the time to do some visualization. I envisioned myself eating healthy clean foods all day, as well as going for a walk at lunch. I pictured myself with each meal, what foods I would choose, the taste and how good it will feel to eat it, as well as how proud of myself I will be at the end of the day after achieving my vision. I imagined myself leaving work at lunch, walking toward the harbour, the buildings I would see on the way there, as well as how beautiful the view is once I reach my destination.

I have never done this before when previously embarking on weight loss programs or healthy eating fads but I did find it to be *a useful tool. My motivation for the day was set in motion once I completed the visualization. This gave me something to refer to for the rest of the day whenever I found myself about to step into my usual habits, for example I would normally go to the food court at lunch and travel from one food place to another to see which fat ingested meal I would be consuming. Whilst eating this meal, I would sit for the whole hour and read while chewing every piece of food on my plate without really realizing it. I get to the end of my lunch and feel as though I haven't eaten anything because it was just mindless, habitual feasting.*

Today this changed.

I decided to go with a boiled egg this morning for breakfast with one slice of wholemeal bread—not sure if this was enough because half-an-hour later I needed a banana and a coffee (which I am trying with one sugar instead of two). I went for the toast and egg so that I could go with fruit for an easy snack at work, and that is what happened.

For morning tea I had a small tub of yogurt with strawberries, it felt really good to eat this as a snack and I had lots of energy until lunch. This is unusual for me as most of the time I would have gone for something easy such as a couple of biscuits with a coffee, a sugary muesli bar, or a muffin. I also skipped the second coffee because it just doesn't go with yogurt and fruit.

I made sure I left the office for lunch and I went for a walk down to the harbour, just as I had imagined. It takes me about twenty minutes to get there and the same back. I then ate a ham and salad sandwich for lunch while sitting in the communal kitchen. I find for some reason it helps me to eat where I know other people can see me as this is a motivational tool for me to be seen eating healthy food (something to mention to Crystal).

By the way, while on my walk I started to think about what I like about myself. My first one is—I like that I am committing to getting healthy.

Once again, I felt full of energy after lunch and I am guessing it was that walk. I don't know why I have never thought of it before as it seems like such an obvious thing to do. Maybe I just associated exercise with a full-on power walk after work with leggings and t-shirt or going to the gym. It didn't occur to me to just bring some comfortable shoes to work and go for a nice walk at lunch—who cares about the pollution!

For afternoon tea I had a handful of almonds, sultanas, craisons and an apple. It felt naughty but I know it isn't. I did go for a cup of tea with this, as I am still in the habit of having a hot drink with snacks.

Before I knew it, it was time to come home. I managed a stir fry with some chicken (the breast) and lots of spinach, broccoli, cauliflower, carrot and celery. I also had half a cup of rice with it.

I still feel like I need something after dinner and I have gone with another suggestion from the handouts—two squares of dark chocolate and I definitely can only go the two squares. That stuff is strong!

Going to bed and still feeling good.

CHAPTER 4

E very morning this week I have taken the time to visualize my day that lies ahead of me, it really has worked in keeping me motivated.

For the rest of the week I pretty much stick to the same foods, alternating from ham and salad sandwiches to cheese and salad sandwiches, with dinner being a small piece of steak with vegetables, or fish and salad, back to chicken and even a meat free evening with lentil and vegetable curry—yum!

I have walked everyday during lunch and if I have to go to another floor in our building I take the stairs instead of the elevator. Once again, all obvious and well known stuff, but I just never applied it before.

The week has gone surprisingly fast considering I am on a . . . . oops, just realized I was falling into that mind trap again. This is not something I am on. It is my lifestyle now and for always. Anyway, the week has gone fast and Saturday has arrived meaning I am due to have my second session with Crystal.

I am a little apprehensive and can't help wondering whether I have lost weight, eaten all the right foods, done enough exercise—just basically done enough all round. In fact this is the first time this week I have had these thoughts and I know it's because I feel my session with Crystal is judgement time, just like all the other meetings with all the other weight loss professionals.

I am glad our meeting time is early this week as I barely managed to eat my breakfast and I am sure my morning stroll along the beach almost worked its way into a run—basically I am nervous and excited about my meeting with Crystal.

I arrive at Crystal's amazing hideaway office and I instantly relax. Maybe I should look at decorating my townhouse like this instead of the boring whites and beige with splashes of blue—a very common combination for safe people. Crystal pops out of the office, interrupting my thoughts. "Morning Ruby" she chirps. "Come on in." I feel really comfortable with Crystal already, almost as if she is one of my dear friends. It doesn't stop the little bit of nerves I have creeping through though.

After a quick chat about the week, Crystal takes a look at my food diary, and before discussing my choices she asks what my feelings were throughout the week with regards to my change in lifestyle.

"I felt really good about it" I say. "I found it interesting that I didn't think about food or what I thought I was missing out on, non-stop like I normally would. I know I am not on a diet, but not eating how I usually would, would be enough to make me depressed and feel deprived. I didn't do that this week. I know it's only early days, but so far so good." I finish up on a positive.

"You are definitely serious and the motivation is there, which is great! I am glad to hear you felt good about your changes Ruby. I think the reason you didn't think about food non-stop was because I didn't place any restrictions on you. I gave you the freedom to choose what you wanted to eat and no one or any piece of paper was telling you otherwise. So before making a choice for each meal, did you stop and think about it?"

"Yes, I did. I thought about what would be nice to eat as well as what I thought would make me feel good and also how it fit into my day."

"And did you at anytime feel deprived?" Crystal asks.

"No. And I'm not sure if that means I did something wrong. Maybe I ate too much or maybe I included foods that aren't as good for me as I thought." I say, not feeling as confident as I did before.

"You haven't done anything wrong, it's not possible, this is your transition into healthy eating, and we will go through your food diary soon so I can help you see this. Also you mentioned before that it is 'early days'. There are no early days Ruby. Don't forget, you are not doing this just to lose weight, with a certain amount of time to achieve this in, you have decided to improve your health, and it has become your lifestyle. The sooner you are able to really understand this, the sooner you are able to feel completely free from your issues with your weight. You want to be fit, and you want to be healthy these are not temporary states for the body, they are where you should always want to be."

So true, so true, so true, I repeat to myself. I know I understand this mentally, but I realize I need to feel it physically and emotionally. It's not easy to change your thought process, but it is possible, it will just take time, I reassure myself.

"Let's discuss your food choices for the week. I see after the first day, you switched to boiled eggs and toast for breakfast, and that is a great choice for during the week. There is protein in there and it is a good substantial breakfast. You could alternate it with a little muesli and Greek Style yogurt, and you could include blueberries if you like them or any other berries of your choice. Greek style yogurt usually has less sugar than even the low-fat ones on the market, as well as being high in good bacteria and protein." Hmm, something I never knew, and I guess I will give it a go, it doesn't sound too bad.

"Sandwiches for lunch are a great easy choice. Lean ham or cheese are good options, you could also choose cottage cheese for something different, maybe some hummus and lots of salad, some turkey and maybe tuna, just to shake it up a little. There is also this great flat bread at the supermarket you can buy which is made mostly out of rice or corn flour, so it has less wheat in it and is low in sugar—this is a good alternative to bread and is tasty. You could also try corn or rice cakes." Oh yes, I had forgotten about those!

"Your choices for dinner are fine too. Don't forget, you could have rice noodles instead of just rice and you could try Quinoa. I am not sure if you like it, but cabbage is a great bulk food and you can cut it to look like spaghetti and have a yummy sauce with vegetables to pour over the top of it." I am not sure about the cabbage, but I am willing to give it a try. If I am going to make the change, there is no point in being shy about it.

"Snacks—the nuts with fruit and even the dried fruit are great. The dark chocolate is a good choice, and if you wanted to you could find a muesli bar that is low in sugar too (there is one on the market that is wheat free and lower in sugar than the others). Just remember to read the tables on the packets. You can buy pre-made popcorn in small packets which are great if you are looking for something different and savoury, maybe not an everyday choice though. Other ideas are celery and carrot sticks with some Tzatziki dip or once again, hummus."

These are all great ideas and some of them, I am sure are on the handouts and I just need to go through them again to remind myself.

"All in all Ruby, I do believe you have made a great start on the path of a healthy lifestyle. Would you mind telling me what you would have normally eaten throughout the week?"

Oh boy! "Well I would usually have cereal for breakfast, something that includes the word bran or flakes with some fruit in it. Then on Friday's which I would consider to be my "special" day, I would get a croissant or a muffin from the patisserie near where I work and take it to my desk with a large latte and eat it there. Lunch would normally have been either a sandwich from the food court or a kebab, Chinese food or something from the Italian take-away, my favourite is their lasagna."

"Dinner usually consists of BBQ chicken from the supermarket with a salad or chips, pasta or rice with vegetables and sometimes meat, a baked dinner for one on Sunday's or sometimes I would just have a bread roll with eggs or even a hamburger from the local take-away. My snacks quite often would be a chocolate bar, biscuits, fruit, and then I always made sure I had dessert which would also be chocolate, ice-cream, custard or cheesecake. One of those, not all of them" I say quickly, just to make sure she didn't think I was a total piggy.

"I didn't eat that stuff all the time but a variety of it throughout the week. Also I know my portion sizes were bigger than they should have been, which reminds me, using the smaller bowl and plate are a great help and a fantastic idea! I realize how much more I was putting on my plate compared to what I really should be eating."

During this confession I expected Crystal to raise an eyebrow, or two. Instead, she sat looking at me with warm eyes that told me she understood. Listing the foods I love, was making my mouth water, as well as giving me some bad ideas for when I leave here. *Stop!* I yell at myself (in my head)—seriously, and is food (and bad ones for that matter) all I can think of? Crystal breaks my thoughts . . . . thank goodness!

"There is nothing wrong with liking all of those foods, it is normal. Coming here to see me is not about getting rid of all those tastes you love either. It's about breaking the habit of having them in your diet so often." *Ha! You said the word diet, I childlishly snigger to myself.* "I know I used the word 'diet'" she says instantly reading my mind again. Crystal is unbelievable, seriously I think she is psychic, or maybe my face is really easy to read, either way, she is good.

"The word 'diet' Ruby has become so misused. People mainly use the word to talk about losing weight when really it describes a way of eating. What you eat daily is your diet, no matter what types of foods are included." Yes, this is true. I mean we all know the true meaning of the word diet but everyone has been so used to attaching it to losing weight, it has become a dirty word that means restrictions.

"I get it" I say. "So we can use the word diet when talking in general about the variety of foods we eat but we are not going to use it in terms of weight loss." She nods to let me know I am on the right track.

"So by letting me know what you love, we can make sure you find a way to include it in your everyday diet. For example, you mentioned hamburgers" she smiles. "There is no reason why you couldn't make your own, once a week. That way you can make sure there is less sodium, no sugar and you can include lots of salad. The same can be done for pizza and kebabs. There are lots of great recipes out there for homemade 'take-away foods' and you choose when to include them, and how often."

"The same can be done for dessert, you can either make a low sugar version at home or you can buy from the supermarket ones that are divided into small serves. If you like ice-cream, then there are plenty available that can be bought in a one serve tub, or a box with 6 or 8 small portions inside. Obviously, everyday can't be full of small portions of junk food but there are ways of fitting in something to help you feel like you aren't restricting or denying yourself anything."

This gives me a lot to think about. I wasn't sure if including even little bits of the things I love was a good idea. I mean would I lose control and have more than I should?

"Small steps Ruby. It's all about taking your time, trusting yourself, and believing that you can take care of your body and your health." She says, reading my mind or it is my face again.

I also go on to ask her about my wanting to eat in the kitchen at work, now that I am eating healthy. "Where would you normally eat your lunch?" she asks. "Usually in a food court," I say. "I always feel self conscious eating in one of those public places. I always feel as though I am being judged by all the people passing by. Whenever I have been on one of my 'diets' I would eat frozen yogurt for lunch, with fruit salad. And even though I knew there was nothing wrong with this choice, I still felt as though people were thinking things like—*there's that fat woman trying to be healthy*, or *who does she think she is kidding, she really just wants to sink her teeth into a big juicy hamburger.* But then it's even worse if I do choose something like a big plate of pasta, or a curry with rice, or worse chips and a burger. Either way, I can't win." I poured my heart out about how I feel when I eat in front of people—anyone. I feel judged no matter where I am or who is watching me.

"Do you really think they are looking at you and your food Ruby?"

"I know they are" I shoot back at her. "Of course they are. They're looking and then they are thinking they know how I got to be this way. They are looking at the overweight woman feasting on fattening junk foods." Now my voice is trembling and I know the tears hanging in my eyes are just seconds away from streaming down my face.

Crystal hands me a box of tissues which I happily take and dab my face with one of them. She is silent, giving me a minute before saying anything. "I bet most of the people aren't thinking anything, you just think they are because you may sometimes feel a little guilty and self-conscious about your choices, as well as being unhappy about how you look. That is why you need to start loving yourself now. Find the things you like about yourself and write them down. Better still, stand in front of the mirror and tell yourself out loud what you like."

"At those times you make the healthier choices, you still feel self-conscious because it is a public viewing of you being aware of your body and trying to make changes, yet the changes haven't happened yet." The people passing by that are judging and thinking things about you that they shouldn't, have no right to because it is none of their business what you eat and how you eat. In order to be successful, you need to stop worrying about what other people think of you and just worry about what you think of yourself. I know it's easier said than done, but work on it, you will get there."

"So do you think you wanting to eat in the kitchen for your colleagues to see, is because you want them to notice you eating healthy food everyday which then helps you to be proud of yourself? Or do you think it may just be a case of you not wanting to be in one of the food courts just yet—it's a safe place to hide."

"Both, I guess. I mean I do want people to notice what I am doing and at the same time I don't want the looks that strangers do give me when I sit down to eat. Also I think if I sit in the kitchen for all to see, then I am less tempted to eat something that would be a bad choice for me."

"You need to stop being so hard on yourself Ruby. Give yourself a chance to settle into the changes you are making and be proud of yourself for doing this. Tell yourself it is ok to have these feelings, and then change your thought into something positive. Because not only are you changing your eating habits, you're also learning to change your thought pattern. You need to break in those new shoes—

remember. They aren't easy to walk in for the first few weeks . . . . ever!" she says with a broad reassuring smile.

"Before you leave, what have you found that you like about yourself."

"I like that I am committing to a healthy lifestyle. I like my smile and I like that I am learning more about myself every day." I say them all with pride and Crystal smiles, acknowledging that I have finally found some wonderful things to say and like about myself.

I leave the session feeling really good and I agree that I need to be easier on myself as well as accept myself for who I am right now at this present moment and not who I want or expect to be in six months or a year from now.

I decide to go for a wander through the new age store and I am feeling very relaxed with a sense of newness glowing around me. I even bought a book about mindfulness. I can't wait to sink my teeth into it and right now I am glad my friends are away for the weekend—no distractions.

Saturday August 11th—12.30am

Dear HJ,

I talked at length today with Crystal, some of the issues I have already written down and some of them I would just rather not go through all over again, therefore I don't feel like putting it to paper, so I will just note down what I have eaten today.

Breakfast—two eggs, baby spinach, tomato and celery— yum! And a cup of tea.

Snack—100g Greek style yogurt with strawberries. I decided to give the Greek yogurt a try as I have been having the low-fat flavoured ones so far. Not sure yet about the yogurt, but I am willing to keep trying it with the strawberries for a while. Half an hour later I had a coffee.

Lunch—4 corn thins with cottage cheese, half an avocado, lots of lettuce, one tomato and lots of cucumber.

Snack—sliced apple, walnuts and a mini pack of sultanas

Dinner—I decide to go all out and make a home—made pizza with a low-fat wrap, chopped tomato, Spanish onion, four olives, pineapple, capsicum (red and green), mushrooms and a light layer of mozzarella cheese. It was delicious and I can't wait to do it again because it is a great weekend meal.

I started reading my book after dinner, so I settled later on with a hot chocolate (one of those sachet ones with low calories).

I was enjoying my book so much I didn't realize it was already midnight. I thought I should really go to bed but I was feeling hungry so I ate a banana. I wouldn't usually eat at this time of night (usually I am asleep of course) and then there have been the times (in the past) when I would go out with my girlfriends, drink a lot and then settle on a kebab before making my way home—I mean, who hasn't done that?

I slowly eat my banana and ponder on what I have been reading so far in my book. I recognize that I do need to change some things in my life. I have let work take over and have fallen into the modern day trap of telling myself I am so busy all the time. I probably say it to other people all the time too, and I am sure they get sick of hearing it. I am busy, but so is everyone else. It is just an excuse. I mean if I am too busy to look after myself, then I have a perfectly good reason to look the way I do or weigh the amount I do. It is such a cop out.

Good night HJ.

Sunday 10.15pm

Dear HJ,

I woke up a little late this morning, at around 8am. I rose feeling fresh and well relaxed. I am not sure if it was my reading material, or all the good food I have been consuming. I like to think it is mostly the latter, but I am sure the book helped too.

I decided on a light breakfast of a beautiful fruit salad topped with Greek yogurt. It was so refreshing and suited the stunning blue sky day that was beaming outside. I then went for a walk to the beach. I walked one way for twenty minutes and sat down so I could read more of my book while sitting on the sand.

I read for an hour, taking in every single minute I was there. I was aware of the sound of the ocean (I have become so used to it. I find it usually falls into the background). I listened to the birds flying over the top of me. People taking dogs for walks, children were splashing and giggling at the shoreline. The sun was warm and the breeze fresh and cold—a perfect day for this time of year.

It felt magical. For the first time ever I was completely relaxed and at peace with myself and my surroundings. I have only been on my healthy life quest for a week and yet I feel better than I ever have and my guess is it can only improve from here on.

I arrived home and decided I should do some cleaning before starting my new week. Even washing clothes and hanging them out to dry seemed better. While hanging the clothes out I actually listened to everything that was happening around me. I could hear the lady next door making a cup of tea. The birds in the tree were chirping so loudly. Do they usually make that much noise? I could hear excited teenagers walking past the block, probably on their way to a café or for a walk to the beach.

How have I not been so awake to what is around me, all this time?

For lunch I had a salad with lettuce, tomato, cucumber, capsicum and some grated carrot. A couple of slices of ham on the side with a little bit of cottage cheese and a light wrap.

I sat in my courtyard and ate lunch so I could continue to take in this perfect day.

After lunch I caught up on some TV that I missed during the week and I had a coffee. I then read for another hour before cooking my dinner.

Dinner—Fish with steamed vegetables. One potato, broccoli, cauliflower, cabbage and carrot.

For dessert I had two pieces of dark chocolate.

I am off to bed early ready for work tomorrow.

Signed Ruby.

CHAPTER 5

I am up early feeling refreshed and ready to face my day. I have a busy one ahead and haven't even had time to think about food but I know I still have to eat healthy and have all my meals as well as snacks. Crystal reminded me that no matter how busy I am it is important for my body to remain nourished and fuelled by good food and water.

I note how right she is as I was aware of how good I felt last week and I am looking forward to experiencing another week just like that.

Monday August 13th

Dear HJ,

What a day! It was full on day at work but I didn't mind because I was still in a good mood from the weekend and I had a lot of energy which kept me going.

I had Greek yogurt, strawberries and wheat free cereal for breakfast, an apple, almonds and coffee for morning tea. For lunch I walked down to the water and bought a salad and chicken wrap (no dressing) from a café. I took the wrap back to work to eat at my desk. For afternoon tea I had a snack pack of rice crackers, a banana and a coffee. I also made sure I drank plenty of water throughout the day.

I got home at about 7.30pm so I put a frozen cannelloni meal (one of those lean ones) into the microwave and it was really nice (I will have to do that more often). Now I am settling down with a cup of hot chocolate to watch a little bit of TV before bed.
   Good night.

It is Saturday morning and I am off to see Crystal again. This will be my third and last weekly visit. From now on I will be going fortnightly on a Thursday night, as she keeps her Saturdays free for new clients. I am glad I get to see her today as I have had a couple of small hurdles throughout the week and I want to make sure I dealt with them the best way possible.

I arrive at her office and as soon as I get there, I feel all the stress from my previous week fade away. I begin to sense all of those emotions that I experienced last week which carried through with me over the weekend and into around Wednesday, which is when it all fell apart.

I only wait about 5 minutes before Crystal's earlier client leaves and she greets me.

"Hi Ruby, how are you today?" she says with a warm smile on her face. "Better, now that I am here" I confess to her. "Sit down and tell me about your week."

"Well, when I left here last week, everything was great . . . ." I go on to tell her about the book I started reading, my lovely weekend where I felt so alive and awake with my senses going wild. I also informed her that my healthy eating was right on track until . . . .

"So I get to Wednesday and I am still feeling great. I am sitting on the bus on my way to work, and I begin to look at the other women on the bus. I am admiring their lovely tight suits and dresses. They fit so nice and snug around their non bulging waistline, all of them had butts that looked like they were hoisted up with fishing line. Necks with no double chins hanging off them and collar bones protruding severely, announcing the thinness of the body they belong to."

"I realized it is going to take me a very long time to get that! I couldn't imagine myself looking like them because I have never been that thin or able to wear those types of clothes. So I got to work and

I was feeling really down, and all I wanted to do was eat a king sized chocolate bar. I could almost taste how good it would feel, to have it in my mouth, the sweetness of it and the smoothness of it around my teeth and tongue. I grabbed my purse and I was heading toward the elevator to go downstairs and a colleague walked by "hi Ruby, you are looking radiant. I don't know what you are doing, but keep it up," she told me I was looking good."

"I turned around, went back to my desk and I called another colleague who I am on friendly terms with and asked her if she could buy me a coffee and bring it to me. I did that so I wouldn't have to go outside and still be tempted." I finished with a big sigh.

"I do know it's difficult" Crystal starts saying, "and I am glad you didn't end up buying a chocolate bar. I wouldn't have been upset with you if you did, but I know that you would have been disappointed with yourself, not because you would have ruined your day, but because the urge to have the chocolate was driven by your emotions. If you can, it is best to save those kinds of foods as treats, not foods to feed your sadness or when you feel stressed. It sounds to me like that colleague was a little bit of divine intervention huh" she says with a compassionate smile.

"It's the same with the other parts of our lives, if we look at what everyone else has then we can never see where we are meant to be. You can certainly use a woman's body that you admire as a visual tool to motivate you to what you hope to get to, but remember the goal is to be and remain healthy, how you end up looking physically, is going to be a bonus."

"Don't try to imagine yourself at that point. Use the visualization tools to imagine yourself being healthy, fit and strong, with no size attached and no ideas of what you are going to wear. I know a lot of people use these as a motivational tool, but it sends a message to your brain that you are only doing the hard work to wear that tiny bikini or those skinny jeans or the little black dress. It needs to be so much more than the physical appearance, so it is important to focus on how you want to feel physically and what you want to achieve for your health too. Remember it is going to continue to be your lifestyle, not a temporary state of being. So what else happened?" she asked.

"After that, I skipped my lunchtime walk and went to the park just across from the office. I spent some time reading my book. You know the one about mindfulness. I felt much better after that and like I had my mind back in the right place." Crystal nods, agreeing that this was a good idea.

"Thursday was all good and I was back to normal. Yesterday, I went out with friends to dinner. We were having a nice chat before it was time to order and I overheard the guy at the table next to us tell his girlfriend not to order the pasta with creamy sauce and garlic bread because he didn't want her to look like the fat lady sitting at the next table. That fat lady was me! I was so embarrassed. When it came to ordering I felt like asking for the creamy pasta, because I began to wonder what I was doing all of this for. I felt like giving up. Why shouldn't I order the fatty dinner on the menu if I really want it. But honestly, it wasn't what I was going to order anyway so I stopped myself. I also didn't want to prove the idiot right, so I ordered the steak with steamed vegetables, like I was intending to in the first place. The funny thing is I couldn't finish the steak. it was quite a big meal. I did decide to share a piece of cheesecake with my friend. I am not sure if that was the right thing to do but I wanted to have it."

"I am sorry about the guy at the other table Ruby. Nothing I say will make that go away. It is amazing how we let people that we don't even know, break our spirit and hurt our feelings. And the cheesecake? It wasn't wrong to share it with a friend, you just found a way to have your cake and eat it too" she says winking and seeming proud of herself for that one.

"Let's do another kind of visualization. This time I am going to guide you through it. You will need to close your eyes and follow my instructions. I will ask you some questions but I want you to answer them to yourself, in your mind—so I can't hear you."

"Close your eyes and relax. I am going to count to twenty and then I want you to relive the moment you just described to me about the bus trip on your way to work. Bring back all those feelings you had, I want you to think them and then physically feel them"

Crystal guides me, and I am back there, on the bus, experiencing the envy I have over all of those young, pretty women with fantastic bodies.

I hear Crystals voice guiding me again. *"Now you are at work, and you decide you want to buy that chocolate bar you felt you needed so much, only this time your colleague doesn't interrupt you. This time, you make it into the elevator and into the shop downstairs. Imagine picking out the perfect chocolate bar that will feed and soothe your emotions. Now pay for it and take it back upstairs to your desk."*

"Look at the packaging, study it and take in the colours that glisten, they are calling your name, inviting you to open it and take your first bite. Smell the chocolate—enjoy the aroma before taking that first bite."

I am there. I am experiencing the all too familiar sensations of giving in to my cravings and holding a chocolate bar in my hands. I continue to follow Crystal's instructions.

"Take your fist bite and chew the piece slowly, then swallow it. Take another bite, and another—keep going until you have finished." She gives me a moment to visualize this.

"Keep your eyes closed and listen to my questions. How did you feel on your way to the shop to buy the chocolate? How did you feel once you paid for the chocolate? What were your thoughts while examining the packaging? How did it feel to take the first bite? How did your mind feel compared to your body while you were eating the chocolate?"

Crystal was pausing for a moment in between questions, allowing me enough time to answer the questions in my mind.

I was asked to continue keeping my eyes closed and sit for a couple of minutes . . . . then one last question—*"And how do you feel now? Physically and emotionally after eating the whole chocolate bar?"*

Crystal counted down and then finally instructed me to open my eyes. This was bizarre, because I felt as though I had really just consumed a chocolate.

"So Ruby, do you mind if we discuss your experience with that" she asks gently. "No not at all" I say.

"Can you recall your answers to the questions, and tell me how you felt?"

"Yes. On the way down to the shop, I felt excited that I was about to buy a chocolate bar because I know how good they taste. At the same time I could feel a tiny bit of anger from my negative thoughts on the bus, as well as sadness and depression brought on by my feelings toward my body and appearance."

"Ok, that's good" she says and I know it's because I have dug deep in search of my emotions.

"When paying for the chocolate, I felt a little self-conscious which is how I normally feel because of the way the assistant looks at me, this then brings on a little bit of guilt, but only drives me to wanting to devour that chocolate bar even more. I am shitty because I like chocolate so why not have a little of it when I want and at the same time, it's like people expect me to like it and they assume I eat a lot of it because of my size."

Crystal's face is intense she is really listening to what I am saying while at the same time looking as though she has experienced this before. "Go on" she says quietly.

"Examining the package, I realized how much I actually do like the look of the wrapper. It glistens like the sun and the packet makes a crisp crinkling sound as I move it around in my fingers. Surprisingly it actually makes it more appealing and I am sure I can smell it before I rip the wrapper open, and I LOVE the aroma of chocolate!" I say with enthusiasm, because I really do.

"The first bit was sensational, as always. I love the feel of the chocolate once it is in my mouth, the way it makes its way around my tongue and teeth, the sweetness, and the gooiness, at the time, there is nothing better in the world. All of my senses are loving the chocolate. I think my body is too, and then the conflict starts. Physically I am feeling as though I should stop, but my mind is saying keep going because the sensations I feel while eating this stuff is just too good. I hate wasting good food, so I eat the whole bar."

Crystal nods in recognition. "And what about afterwards?" she asks. "As soon as I finish the chocolate, I still feel good and I want more. It's like I could keep going, and I want to go and buy another bar. Within five to ten minutes though, it hits me. I feel fat, bloated, guilty, tired, cranky and disappointed that I gave in to the craving or the emotional battle I was having in my mind that led me to getting the chocolate in the first place."

"That was really good Ruby. I can tell you are using your visualization exercises frequently by the way you responded to this activity. Doing this gave you the ability to see further into yourself and how you feel once giving in to a craving or your emotional eating. You can now refer to this exercise and grab the feelings you experienced during it next time you feel yourself slipping into an old habit. This is a very strong tool to have for any challenges that pop up and I am sure there will be plenty more along the way. It will get easier though as your new habits form and just become a way of life."

"I also want you to be aware that you are in mourning"

"Mourning, for what?" I manage to squeak. "For you" she says. "You are changing from the woman who always used food for comfort and your extra weight as a shield, to now facing your emotions and challenges, and tackling them head on." She left it at that. No more explanation needed. She was right and I knew it. I came to know food as something that would fit and feed all of my emotions.

When I was stressed, I munched on chips. The sound and motion of the crunching soothed my nerves. For sadness or if I felt depressed I turned to chocolate and sometimes ice-cream, depending on the time of day I felt it, but usually chocolate. When I am happy, which really is most of the time I just eat whatever looks good. And then there were the routine foods—the ones for reading, watching TV or a good movie at night and the ones to have with tea and coffee . . . . oh and I mustn't forget the social foods. They are all things from cakes, biscuits, chocolate, ice-cream, chips, dip and crackers.

I never sat at home constantly eating junk food. I always believed I ate healthy foods but it was different. For example I would eat cereal for breakfast (one of the "healthy kind") but I now know I put too much in the bowl, this meant extra milk too. I ate fruit, but I also managed to always add a cookie here and there or chocolate but I would have one at morning tea, then one or two after lunch, and so on. I always had healthy food in my diet, but I also made sure I comforted myself with all the other stuff.

I do hide behind my weight. I got so big I became used to the idea that this is the way I am meant to stay, so I have always made sure I did. Sub-consciously I knew that looking this way meant it was harder to meet new people, men or women. If I didn't meet them, then they didn't have the chance to dump me as a friend or lover once they decided I was too fat for them.

"So you did say you were having a great week though" Crystal interrupts my deep thoughts. "You mentioned how you were in a good head space. How did you feel physically?"

"I had a lot of energy" I recall with a big smile of my face. "I still do. And I feel lighter when I walk. My thinking is clearer and I am less stressed, even though I had a huge week at work. I know it's only been two weeks and I keep wondering if it is possible to feel this good so soon. I mean, with all the programs I have followed in the past I never felt this good."

"Why do you think that is" Crystal asks. "I believe it is because even though I haven't eaten certain foods, I actually haven't told myself I can't eat them. I did stop myself from buying the chocolate bar and ordering the creamy pasta but it was for a different reason. I instinctively knew I wanted those foods due to me being emotional. Therefore, I was aware I was going for them for all the wrong reasons.

At other times, when it has crossed my mind to have something I know is not the healthiest option, I have just simply asked myself, *how is this food helpful in me becoming healthy?* Or, *is this going to benefit my body nutritionally?* I didn't even think about weight loss, and of course my answer to both those questions was that it won't help my health, and it isn't nutritional for me" I sat there quite proud of my thought process and I became aware of how much progress I am making.

"You are well on your way Ruby. Keep all of those good feelings and questions close to you so you can grab them when you need to. We can't eat healthy foods 100% of the time, it's unrealistic. It is all about balance, moderation and not placing limitations on yourself so that your choices are based on what your body needs and not what your eyes see, and think you want or need. So Ruby, what have you discovered you like about yourself this week."

"I like that I became aware of that fact that my emotions wanted to be fed and I didn't give in to them. I like the way I am feeling physical and mentally from following a healthy lifestyle. I like my hands. They are always thin when the rest of my body isn't."

We both laugh at this, and Crystal tells me I am doing a great job at looking within and discovering likeable things about myself. I have to admit, doing this exercise is helping me to like who I am and I am on my way to loving Ruby.

Our time has come to an end and I am grateful for this session as well as feeling emotionally drained. I feel I have let a lot out as well as waking up to some of my deeper feelings.

CHAPTER 6

I get home and eat a fruit salad for a snack. It felt so fitting considering I had just let some emotional toxins expel from my mind and body. I follow that with a walk to and along the beach, I needed to fill myself with some renewed energy.

I arrive home refreshed and I am really looking forward to my salad with low fat cheese and a wrap. A few minutes after finishing lunch my friend Michelle is calling my mobile. "Hi, how are you?" I say happy she has rung. "Good! Hey how about coming to a barbeque this afternoon, it starts at around 4pm." I hesitate, she pushes a little and then I give in and agree to go with her. "Great, I will pick you up around 3.45pm."

Damn it! I didn't want to go. The females will be there in their tight jeans, body hugging jumpers, knee high boots, flattering fitted jackets. I catch myself falling into that mind trap again. I let the thoughts go and I remind myself that this harsh self talk is not constructive at all. This is what I have always done. Find a positive now—I like to socialize and I can't do that sitting in my lounge room watching TV alone.

I tell myself to forget about my physical appearance and to go out for a chat and a laugh. That is what meeting up with people is all about. It isn't for strutting your stuff like a show pony. But of course there will be men there ogling the glamour pusses but I need to forget about that because a man is not on my list of priorities at the moment anyway. They can have the other women that will be there. I am going out purely for some fun.

I dig out a wrap dress that looks great with the knee high boots I own (not the ones with the zips up the side, they don't fit—these are the stretch ones). I always receive compliments when I have worn this dress, it sits well on my curves and the colours suit my complexion. I put it on and I am surprised it is a little loose on me! The good thing is I can adjust it to fit and I am smiling to myself and feeling very pleased. I guess I have lost some weight. I am glad I threw out my scales otherwise I would have been tempted to weigh myself. I still wouldn't have been happy with the number, but I am impressed with the looseness of the dress and how it looks.

It is 3.45pm and I walk out the door with confidence.

Midnight—Saturday

Dear HJ,

What a day! I had two scrambled eggs for breakfast with grated carrot and zucchini. A fruit salad for morning tea, and a salad with low fat cheese in a wrap for lunch.

I was invited to a barbeque, so I saved my afternoon snack for when I got there. I took a packet of rice crackers and a jar of salsa for the party but of course made sure I was close enough to it so I wouldn't have to eat anything else. I took a piece of chicken breast to cook on the barbeque and someone else brought a salad. I shared a bottle of wine with my friend but we only had two standard glasses each. After dinner someone put a box of chocolates on the table so I had two and then I walked over and sat by the pool until they were ravished by everyone else.

I had such a great night even though I didn't want to go. I only knew a couple of people and the rest I was meeting for the first time. All the women were nice and not all of them were roaming around in tight outfits, in fact one or two of them weren't exactly skinny, not that that should make a difference. And the guys there were lovely and capable of an intelligent conversation. I am not sure if it is because I was feeling more confident, therefore I was more open to everyone talking to me.

I need to go to bed because it is very late.

10pm—Sunday

Dear HJ,

I had a really nice day. I woke up a little later than usual from my late night, but it felt good to have a lazy morning. I had Greek yogurt and fruit for breakfast and because it was late, I didn't need anything else until lunch.

For lunch I had tuna salad and a wrap. I munched on some rice crackers and a hand full of almonds for afternoon tea and for dinner I decided to make myself a homemade hamburger. It was really yummy, better than what I would have bought from the local take away.

I went for a walk but it wasn't very long. It was only 10 minutes down the road and back to get the Sunday paper.

I read for the rest of the afternoon but feel I needed it after last week.

It is Monday morning again and I am looking forward to tackling this week. I also find myself thinking about my previous adventures of trying to change my body and how I have always been told that after 21 days of following any new routine or habit it is easier to follow through with it and then stick to it from then on.

At the end of this week, it will be 21 days since I had my first appointment with Crystal and I am trying not to think about it. I agree that this is completely different to previous plans where my primary goal was to lose weight, but I am still changing many habits as well as training my brain to take a different approach although, I feel this is happening bit by bit as the days are passing.

I have had my shower and without thinking, I start chopping strawberries and washing grapes, I then grab the yogurt from the fridge and top it all with a handful of wheat free muesli. This has become my habitual before-work-breakfast and I am really enjoying it.

It is such a beautiful morning I decide to leave home 15 minutes earlier than I usually do. The bus stop closest to my place is only two minutes away, so I decide to walk to the next one (which only took me another 8 minutes), so I thought I would risk it and get to the next bus stop. I made it just in time for the bus. I really pushed myself making sure I didn't miss it. I was puffed out when I sat down and to be honest I was a little embarrassed, hoping the other passengers didn't think it was just from me climbing the three steps into the vehicle.

I arrive at work to find I have totally forgotten about a meeting that was scheduled. All is good because the paperwork I need to present to my boss is all done which is a sigh of relief. I walk into the boardroom and of course there is a whole lot of food staring at me from the table along the back wall. There are cupcakes with pretty, fluffy pink and white icing, croissants with melted ham and cheese, blueberry muffins, doughnuts and some Danish scroll things.

It is ok, I begin telling myself, *I can cope with this because I am not on a diet and I am not denying myself anything, I am aware that none of this food is beneficial to my health therefore, I choose not to eat it.*

I sit feeling very proud of myself and the success of my self-talk. "Hi Ruby!" It's Jenny from downstairs. Great! She is quite overweight and (like me) always on a diet but when we have these meetings she tries at least one thing from each plate and makes me do it with her (maybe make isn't the right word but she is very persuasive, and so is the food). "Come and join me at the food table" she says with a big salivating grin on her face. The truth is while it all looks yummy—I really just don't feel like it. I was actually looking forward to my rice crackers and banana this morning.

Oh, what to say . . . . what to say . . . . "Hi Jenny, I don't think I will this morning I uh, had the runs before I left this morning. It seems to have subsided a little, (I whispered) but I can't be quite sure, I still have some cramping in my stomach." "Eew," she says looking at me like I just exploded right in front of her. "Yes might be best not to eat any of that stuff. Don't pass it on to me!"

"You better stay right away from me then." I say brushing her off with my hand.

I have never lied to get out of eating before, but I know she would have just kept on at me if I had just said 'no'.

The meeting dragged a little longer than I expected and my stomach was beginning to rumble. I am sure everyone could hear it. I did receive some pretty weird looks from the others in the room. I think they thought I was going to start gnawing off parts of their bodies.

I excused myself to "go to the ladies room" and all nodded except for Jenny. She gave me that 'I feel your pain sympathetic look'. Feeling a little guilty, I ran to my office and gobbled down the banana I had at my desk. I was so hungry, it had to be done.

I quickly get back to the meeting and at least my hunger has disappeared for the meantime but I know myself well enough to know it will be back in about thirty minutes.

The meeting finishes and I am able eat the rest of my snack, and continue my day as normal.

Monday—9.30pm

Dear HJ,

Breakfast today was the usual. I had a meeting at work and lied to a co-worker to get out of eating junk food. I think it is kind of funny because three weeks ago I would never even given it a thought (lie to get out of eating). I made it through and ate my banana and rice crackers for morning tea and I managed to sneak in a coffee.

At lunch I went for a walk (oh yeah, I got in about 15 minutes walk this morning too), so all up today I got around one hour of exercise. I made myself a really nice wrap with salad and a small can of four bean mix for lunch.

For a snack this afternoon I had a cup of tea and two slices of cheese, some almonds, walnuts and sultanas.

47

Dinner was chicken breast, one medium sized potato, cauliflower, broccoli, carrot and green beans.

After dinner I had two pieces of dark chocolate.

Good night and looking forward to some yummy healthy food tomorrow.

Tuesday 8pm

Dear HJ,

Another great day. I ate my usual breakfast of Greek yogurt with fruit and muesli, lunch was tuna with salad and some corn thins, I had carrot and celery sticks for both morning and afternoon tea, with some sultanas. I also had a cup of tea and two coffees and it is normal for me to have one sugar now instead of two. For dinner, I decided to give tofu a try and made it as a stir fry with vegetables. It was really good!

My mum rang me today and mentioned we hadn't seen each other for a few weeks. Which is true, I haven't been avoiding her, just a little busy. She is coming over with Emmy on Saturday for morning tea. This is good, because I can make something healthy so my changes won't be obvious to her. It's not that I don't want her to know about my lifestyle change, it's just that she will go on at me about how I have tried too many diets with none of them working and I just end up being disappointed and frustrated with myself. I really couldn't be bothered yet to try and explain to her how this is different, I would rather her see the changes for herself.

I am just about to eat a single serve ice-cream and watch a movie, and then it will be off to bed for me.

CHAPTER 7

Saturday August 25th

Saturday has arrived and I have been scanning and studying any recipes I have from the health magazines Crystal gave me, plus a couple more I have acquired along the way. I have settled on Carrot and Apple Bran muffins, I quite like the sound of them.

It very quickly makes its way to 10am. Mum and Emmy are knocking at my door. "Yum, it smells good in here" my mum says as soon as I let them in. "That will be the muffins I have just pulled from the oven" I say with pride. "Here is a cake from the patisserie you love so much." Great! That is all I need, a reminder of my past Saturday routine. *All is good,* I say to myself, *I can cope with this.*

The coffee smells good, and we are soon sitting down enjoying our morning tea. Then mum starts asking me if I have "found anyone suitable yet?" Really! Does she have to go through this every three months, it is annoying enough that I think about it, I don't need her constantly questioning me.

"No mum, no one has appeared on the horizon yet" I say with slight annoyance in my tone of voice. "I only want you to be happy Ruby. Don't get upset with me for asking." Oh, no, maybe I was too harsh with her. "I am happy mum. Thank you for your concern. I am just concentrating on myself at the moment and work."

"Well, you are looking healthy, but work won't always be there for you, you know." I ignore the last comment but smile recalling her comment about how I am looking healthy. She has never given me a compliment like that before.

Emmy is her usual chirpy self, trying to change the conversation every time she notices it getting awkward between me and mum. To be honest I am glad I have a sister and I prefer it when it is the three of us, it means I can usually sidestep more questions my mother has for me. We do get along, it's just that she never gives up about me finding a man, and it does get annoying. I know she loves me and just wants the best for me.

Our time together has come to an end, it has been fun (kind of). Emmy tells me how much she loved the muffins so I manage to talk her into taking the rest home.

I decide to go for a walk to the beach after lunch. It is a beautiful day and I can smell spring in the air even though it is not quite here yet. Lots of people are out and about. Picnics are being held on the grass, children are playing in the park, there are people dining in the restaurants and cafes that capture the gorgeous view of the water across the road. It is busy and all of a sudden, I realize I don't want to be alone tonight.

I fetch my phone out of my purse and ring Michelle to invite her over to my place tonight, she accepts and volunteers to phone the other girls for me so I can continue my walk. I am feeling satisfied knowing that I will not be experiencing a lonely Saturday night in front of the TV.

Now I am wishing I kept some of those muffins to give the girls for dessert. What am I thinking! They just would've made fun of me anyway, trying to serve them muffins for dessert, especially healthy ones. I text Michelle and ask her to pick something up on the way.

Six o'clock arrives and so do Michelle, Nat, Sam and Danni. We all agree on Thai food for dinner which is easy for me because I am not exactly great at cooking for one, let alone four other people. I think they were all secretly relieved too that I wasn't doing the cooking.

The wine is open and the night is flowing. I decide that I am not going to be too concerned about my alcohol consumption for the evening. I am not usually a big drinker, although I have had my moments so I am confident I will have what I need and not a drop more.

"So, I see you have given the health kick the flick!" cheers Danni. "No" I respond, "I am continuing to eat healthy, and I feel great, so there is nothing to give the flick to." "Really" she says, and laughing annoyingly. "Why are you drinking and pigging out on rice crackers and dip?" Not that it is any of her business, but I answer her anyway. "Firstly, I am allowed to drink and eat whatever I like. Secondly I am not pigging out, I am eating and drinking in moderation and have been for the last few weeks. You should try it sometime" Maybe the last sentence shouldn't have left my mouth but I couldn't help it, she does this to me every time. She looked a bit shocked and hurt . . . . everyone was quiet.

"Oh well, whatever! I just don't see how you can lose weight eating like that" Eating how? Healthy? In moderation? Not like I used to? All of these questions, or statements rather were what I felt like saying to her but instead I just responded as politely as I could. "Danni, I am not on a diet or trying to lose weight, I am eating as healthy as I can in order to feel better and it is working. If I happen to lose weight while doing it, then I consider it a bonus." I left it at that.

Later, after I calmed down, I realized that her reaction was probably due to the fact that she isn't yet ready for the path I have taken and she is feeling jealous, envious or maybe intimidated . . . . whatever her emotion, it led her to lashing out at me because now I am not on her level anymore. I am not saying I am above her or better than her but she may be feeling left out because she used to consider me as the same as her and I too felt comfortable that someone in our group was just like me, but I am over that. I want to be healthy and feel healthy—for me. And for once, I am achieving that.

Saturday 1.30am

Dear HJ,

I was going to skip this entry because it is so late and I am tired, but I decided to take the five minutes needed to write about my day.

I started this morning with fruit salad because my mum and sister were coming for morning tea and I knew I would indulge a little, which I did. I made 'healthy muffins' which honestly were a little sweet for my liking. What the?? Did I just write 'they were a little sweet for my liking' hmm, I am shocked because nothing has ever been too sweet for me. Anyway, next time I think I will half the sugar that is in the recipe . . . . now that is really strange, I think I am really tired!

I also ate a little bit of the cake my mum bought from the Pattiserie. I loved eating it at the time but it was extremely sweet and not long after having it, I wondered why I had bothered—recalling the visualization experience from my visit with Crystal, I now understand exactly how to use it in the future.

I wasn't extremely hungry for lunch after mum and Emmy left, so I made myself a garden salad and ate a slice of ham. I then went for a walk to the beach and back, which was about 45 minutes.

My friends came over for dinner. I ate some rice crackers and tomato salsa, had some red wine and Thai for dinner. I ordered a green curry with vegetables and tofu. I didn't have any rice or noodles with it. I honestly didn't need to because the meal was really filling.

Michelle bought fruit and ice-cream for dessert. I love her! She knows how committed I have been to eating healthy and she bought the fruit because she knew I could eat it and the ice-cream for the others who aren't on their healthy eating quest. I decided that because I had a muffin and some cake this morning, I would go with just the fruit for dessert, which was beautiful and refreshing after the Thai food.

The night was fun, even though Danni caused a bit of a stir, but we were all good after our little conversation about my current food habits and I think I could see her mind ticking after it. Maybe she will seriously consider doing this for herself, but of course it is completely up to her.

I drank about half a bottle of wine, which is the most I have had in a while and I felt it. In saying that, it is off to bed for me. Goodnight HJ, I love you ☺

Sunday 8.30pm

Dear HJ,

I woke this morning feeling a little worse for wear. I wasn't hung over but I did drink more than I have in about a month and I couldn't sleep very well. So, a lack of sleep and a bit to drink and that was it for me. I must be getting old or maybe this healthy lifestyle is kicking in and I am now sensitive to any changes to my diet and lifestyle.

My body must have been screaming out for protein because from the moment I woke up I felt the need to have eggs for breakfast. So I whipped up a really good batch of scrambled eggs, with spinach, carrot, onion and celery in it and I had a slice of wholegrain toast. It was soooo good!

I have made real progress, because back in the old days after a late night with some wine, I would have been down at a certain food chain ordering a big breakfast with coke, now just the thought of it actually makes me feel ill.

I had a tuna salad for lunch and another 45 minute walk to the beach. I grabbed the paper, came home, made a coffee and read the paper for a while. Wow! I can't believe how quickly this weekend has gone.

For dinner I made vegetarian lasagna, it was yummy. It was made with broccoli, cauliflower, tomato puree and cottage cheese with lasagna sheets of course. I had never made it like this before, but I will be making it again. I even have some left for tomorrow night—easy dinner!!

No need for an after dinner snack, because I am off to bed for an early night. Hopefully I can sleep tonight.

CHAPTER 8

It has been nearly four months since I started on my healthy eating lifestyle. I have to admit, I feel fantastic! My skin looks the best it ever has, the whites in my eyes are white (not off white or yellow), and I have more energy than I have had in my whole life. To be honest, it hasn't been easy getting to this point but I am extremely proud of myself, because now my healthy lifestyle is just a part of who I am and I have learnt a lot along the way.

There is a bonus, as Crystal mentioned . . . . I have lost some weight. People have noticed! I haven't stood on the scales to see what my new number is, as I am not ready to do that yet. I am guessing if I was losing weight consistently throughout the three months, then I would probably have lost around 10-15 kilos. It doesn't sound like a lot, but it is to me and that is why I feel right now the number is not the best visual motivation for me. Something that is motivational is the fact that I have gone down a couple of dress sizes and I am ecstatic with this progress. I am pulling out old clothes from my wardrobe to wear, and when I am much smaller, I will have to go shopping as I have never been in a smaller dress size than this before.

I am still enjoying my consultations with Crystal, she always keeps me on the right track when I start to fall back into old thought patterns, or doubt myself. She never tells me what to do and she always seems to find a way to make me aware of my issues on my own, like a light bulb moment.

I am also excited because I am going away for the weekend tomorrow with Michelle, Sam and Nat. Danni couldn't make it for some reason. Whatever it was, it just sounded like a lame excuse, but who am I to judge. I guess it is a good enough reason to her.

This is our pre-Christmas get away get together. We try to do it every year. Sometimes we book a really posh restaurant and dress in formal wear for the evening and then stay in a hotel in the city for the night. Another time we just spent the day at a Spa and had a totally relaxing day with bubbles and chocolate and pampering. So this year we are travelling a couple of hours up the coast and staying in a house for two nights.

It's Friday morning, and we head off for our weekend away. It is nice to have the day off work, and even though we are coming back Sunday afternoon, I took the liberty of asking for Monday off as well, just to get over my weekend away.

I made sure I had my hearty scrambled egg with veggies breakfast, so I wouldn't want anything other than a coffee when the girls stop at one of the take away chains. It worked. All I needed was that good old coffee.

We arrive at the house and we need to go shopping for food, but first dropping off all our luggage is a priority because, well there is four women and yes, we each packed a lot for just two days.

Upon entry to the house I am impressed and I instantly wish this was my home. There are four bedrooms upstairs, two with an ensuite each and walk-in robes. The house is high on a hill and there is a panoramic view of the ocean—'oh beautiful!' And every room in the house has this view. A gourmet kitchen with its own coffee machine! There is a sensational deck for us to wine and dine on and an oversized living area with a large flat screen TV. This is going to home and heaven for the weekend.

We pile into the car to buy our food for the next couple of days. On the way, we discuss whether to go to a restaurant tonight or tomorrow night. Decisions, decisions! We decide on eating out tomorrow night being a Saturday and tonight will be a BBQ on the deck.

We purchase everything from fruit, vegetables, meat, bread, eggs, milk, chips, dips, chocolate and ice-cream. At this point, I am not worried about what I am going to eat because as you can see, we have something for everyone. Being the holiday enthusiasts we are we also place some Christmas decorations in the trolley for us to put around the house. It is after all our own little Xmas party weekend.

We get back to the house and our weekend away is off to a good start!

CHAPTER 9

Sunday 9pm

Dear HJ,

I haven't written in my journal since Thursday night. I left early on Friday morning for a weekend away with friends. I had a fantastic time!

Friday morning, I made sure I ate a really good scrambled egg with veggie breakfast. I had coffee on the way up the coast. I also took a banana with me so I had a snack for the car ride.

For lunch we made a big salad and bought a BBQ chicken from the supermarket. I ate some of the breast with no skin and a large amount of salad. We bought a lot of fruit so I had a fruit salad for my afternoon snack, and a handful of almonds. For dinner we had steak and vegetable skewers done on the BBQ. The skewers were sensational. After dinner I had a single serve ice-cream. I drank two glasses of wine over the whole night, and before dinner we had some nibbles on the table, so I ate some rice crackers and tomato salsa.

I was really pleased with myself for still being able to include my healthy eating while being away. I guess it helped staying in a house and being able to buy and cook our own food.

Saturday was a slightly different story . . . . unfortunately. The day started really well, with me waking up quite early and going for a walk along the beach. It was a ten minute walk down the hill that the house is perched on, so I wasn't really looking forward to the walk back—but I know I need to push myself more when it comes to exercise therefore I knew I had to do it. The beach is gorgeous and I walked along it for about 40 minutes. By the time I arrived back at the house, I was completely puffed from my struggle back up the hill and as red as a beetroot. I had a shower and felt better for taking the opportunity to get some exercise in. Breakfast was out on the deck, with a beautiful fruit salad and some Greek yogurt.

This was the perfect opportunity for me to take in the amazing colours of the fruit in my salad, and take in the high energy they, that is about to replenish my body with nutrients. The colours in the fruit are so vibrant—taking in the greens, yellow, reds and orange, I am grateful I have access to this amazing food group.

We drove in to town at about 9.30am and had a look around the lovely boutiques the village has to offer. We decided it was time for some morning tea and we found a lovely beachside café with amazing views. I ordered scones with jam and asked them not to include the cream. I am pretty pleased with my choice, because scones are definitely healthier than cheesecake, mudcake, sticky date pudding, or banana cream pie. The coffee was really good too.

We stayed in town and made a dent in our pockets by continuing our shopping. Retail therapy felt good! Nat suggested we get some takeaway and sit on the grass at the Mariner for lunch which we did. We ordered fish and chips, it tasted so good in my mouth, I didn't want to stop eating it. I did find I became full quite soon after eating and had to stop before everyone else.

Within 15 minutes of stopping I felt horrible. I was aware of the film the oil had left on my lips and inside my mouth. I was beginning to feel bloated and really lethargic like I didn't want to get up and move from the grass. I don't ever remember feeling like this after eating fish and chips in the past but then again maybe I was so used to feeling this way, I never noticed it. Unfortunately, it's not possible to avoid take-away for the rest of my life, but I guess I could have taken a look around to see if there were any better *options for me, instead of going for the first thing I saw. At least I know if I crave take-away when I don't need it, I can recall these feelings for future reference to avoid giving in to the craving.*

We headed home with our purchases and then headed to the beach for some lazing on the sand. I was a bit hesitant to go to the beach because I have never felt comfortable in a swimsuit but with some positive self talk, I managed to get myself there. Once we settled on the sand, I took a look around and noticed so many other women walking comfortably in their swimmers. They were all shapes and sizes, some nice and slender (of course) and others slightly overweight, some bigger than me and women around the same size as me. If they were self conscious about their bodies, they didn't show it. I quickly became aware that it is me who is uncomfortable with the way I look and not other people around me. Then, for the first time ever, I was quite content with my body and how I look because I know that I eat healthy and I am taking care of myself and I think it is actually showing.

Guess I can now honestly tell Crystal that I like my body, no matter what it looks like.

Three hours after lunch I was starting to feel a little better but still slightly uncomfortable inside somewhere . . . . it is hard for me to explain it.

It was time to get ready for our evening out. While making up our faces and styling our hair, we sipped on champagne and nibbled on crackers and cheese. I got carried away with the night and didn't think about my eating habits. No deprivation and no diet, so there was no need to—I was having fun.

We arrived at the swish restaurant situated at the Mariner overlooking the waterfront, and ushered to our table located out on the balcony. Soon after, the wine was flowing. We ordered a seafood platter for the four of us which came with chips. Not chips again! I just ate them for lunch—anyway . . . . I ate lobster, prawns, fish fried in batter, calamari rings, there was definitely no room for any chips even if I had so desired.

We sat talking for an hour after dinner, when someone mentioned dessert. Even though all four of us moaned we couldn't fit anything else in our stomachs, none of us could resist dessert in this amazing restaurant with its fine dining menu. We decided on a dessert platter to share which consisted of mini cakes and slices—it was perfect, because I could only put two tiny servings into my body.

I woke the next morning feeling a little hung over even though I didn't think I had drunk too much . . . . it must have been the champagne we consumed before leaving the house. I wondered if I should go for a walk to the beach, I couldn't be certain I would make it back up the hill especially the way I was feeling. I decided to leave it and went in search of some fruit, my body was craving it. I found what was left—a couple of bananas, strawberries and grapes. That was enough for me to combine with some yogurt for breakfast. A big coffee was also in order too.

By lunchtime, I found I was salivating at the thought of a light fresh salad, never before has this happened to me. Luckily there was still plenty left and I made a big batch for everyone. I had tuna with mine while everyone else opted for ham or chicken.

At 1.30pm it was time to leave which was a shame. The weekend went way too fast and I am thanking myself for planning ahead and asking for tomorrow off. I arrived home at around 4pm and while I enjoyed myself, I was also happy to be able to get back into my normal routine.

I realized I didn't have a lot of food in the fridge or pantry so I decided on scrambled eggs for dinner. I had to cook frozen vegetables to have with it because I didn't have any fresh ones in the house. I am glad I had some potatoes so I cooked one to include in my veggie mix.

I am going to watch TV now.

Monday 10pm

Dear HJ,

I fell asleep watching TV last night. I somehow made it to bed in the early hours of the morning and I woke up at a nice

7.30am. I really did leave myself short in the food department because I didn't even have anything suitable for breakfast, except for eggs but I had that for dinner last night and I didn't really feel like it for breakfast.

I needed something fast so I walked to the cafes down the road and chose the one with fruit and yogurt on its menu. The fruit was great but I am not sure what kind of yogurt they use because I found it to be really sweet. It was labeled as vanilla on the menu and I am now used to plain yogurt.

I sat thinking about my weekend away. I am really proud of the fact that I have formed a lot of new habits, and going away for the weekend helped me to realize it. I haven't had take-away for ages so when I did eat it, it didn't take long for me to feel horrible afterwards. The last half of Saturday consisted of me consuming large amounts of food I don't eat anymore and by Sunday I was craving all the healthy foods I am now used to. Going away was a real eye opener for me and it is proof that I have overcome bad habits and formed good ones that are here to stay.

I desperately needed to go shopping for food and loved my visit to the fruit and vegetable store where I could see all those brightly coloured healthy foods quickly filling up my trolley. A quick dash to the grocery store to bulk up on my wheat free muesli, Greek yogurt, cottage cheese, rice cakes and corn thins, lean meats and a little bit of dark chocolate for those cravings. I couldn't wait to get home to have my ham and salad wrap.

After lunch I went for an hour's walk. While I was out I got thinking about my exercise, instinctively, I feel I am not doing enough anymore. The walking is a lot easier for me than it used to be and I am wondering if I need more. More walking that includes hills? Or maybe something else to include with my walks, you know, alternate my days with walking and . . . . something.

I am thinking a personal trainer, but at the same time I don't want to let my mind take me to that place. A personal trainer would mean more work—physically. God I am so lazy. Or is it just that I don't think I am at that level yet. I don't believe I would be able to cope with that kind of physical activity. I pondered it while out walking and decided I would talk to Crystal about it when I see her on Thursday this week.

For my afternoon snack I had some almonds, sultanas, an apple and a coffee. I felt the need to give meat a rest, so dinner was my favourite tofu and curry vegetable dish. While I was cooking it, I couldn't wait for it to be ready. Most surprising was while I was chopping the cauliflower and broccoli, my mouth was watering! OMG, there is something wrong with me. No there isn't—but I am giggling at the thought of it because I never thought it was possible for your mouth to water at the site of broccoli or cauliflower. I think too it was my body screaming out for the all vitamins and minerals my dish had to offer after a semi non-nutritious weekend.

I am feeling good. I am a beautiful, healthy person.

CHAPTER 10

Thursday early evening has arrived and I am waiting to be greeted by Crystal. I am excited because I feel like I am at a real turning point in my life and I can't wait to share it with my healthy lifestyle coach.

We are sitting in the consulting room and Crystal has asked me how things have been since our last meeting. "Great!" I say, and then continue to tell her how my weekend went—food and all.

"Wow" she says, "sounds like you had a really good time Ruby." I nodded enthusiastically. "So, you told me how you felt physically after eating the take away, the nibbles before going out and the restaurant meal, but how did you feel mentally and emotionally. For example, were you disappointed? Or did you feel as though you had ruined your healthy eating regimen? Or maybe you didn't feel either of those, maybe you are comfortable with going outside of your normal eating routine now."

I had to think about this for a minute. "I regretted Saturday for a short time, only because of how I felt physically, not because I was worried about ruining anything" I say to her. "Even though I didn't like the way I felt physically, I knew it wasn't worth beating myself up over it. When I had time to think about the weekend, I knew that most of the time, I had managed to stick to the healthy foods I wanted and needed. Also because my mission is to eat and maintain a healthy body, I wasn't worried about slipping up and it affecting my weight.

I am in it for the nutritional benefits, not to shed kilos fast and then scold myself because I may have put on a few hundred grams."

Crystals face brightened and I could sense her excitement. "Ruby, that is fantastic! You are well and truly following a healthy lifestyle. Those new shoes are definitely on the comfortable side right now and are happily walking along the path. I knew you were committed to your healthy lifestyle, but what you just said to me, shows that you now really understand it and are living it. I am extremely happy for you."

She weighs me and still has a wide smile on her face, so I am not sure if that means I have put on weight, lost it or stayed the same. But it doesn't matter because I feel healthy and I am improving my fitness by the day. That reminded me that I needed to ask her if she thought I could do with a program through a personal trainer.

She agreed that it could be a good thing as it would boost my motivation for continuing with my healthy lifestyle and obviously help to improve my fitness levels. I voiced my concerns about not being fit enough to cope physically with this kind of exercise. Crystal suggested I could use the visualization techniques I have been using so far for my walking, but to now imagine myself exercising with a trainer and building up my fitness and strength. Sounds like a good idea to me! She then gave me a business card with a trainer's name and number on it, plenty of Crystal's other clients have worked with her and loved it, so I said I would give her a call.

Friday December 7th, 10.30pm

Dear HJ,

For breakfast this morning I had strawberries, Greek yogurt, grapes and wheat free muesli. For morning tea I made a coffee, and I hadn't had a snack yet, as I really felt like a cookie. I went to the communal kitchen, and surveyed the selection sitting in the jar. I had my head bent nearly all the way into the jar staring at them—they look good. I imagined myself taking a couple back to my desk and enjoying them with my coffee. It didn't take long for it to dawn on me, that I would be disappointed after eating the cookies because really, it is just a whole lot of sugar. I would just be consuming empty calories, so all I would get from eating them, is two minutes of pleasure—nothing else. My stomach would probably rumble within fifteen minutes, because I didn't eat real food that was nutritionally beneficial to me and able to feed and sustain my hungry body.

I happily placed the jar back onto the bench, and I walk away standing tall.

So instead, I ate a handful of mixed nuts, sultanas (a mini pack) and two squares of dark chocolate, with my coffee—a much better choice I think.

At lunch I went for my usual walk, which once again reminded me I needed to make that phone call to the personal trainer. Guess I am a little hesitant to call because I am a bit scared. It's silly because I really feel the need to increase my activity in order to build my fitness levels. I don't want to get to forty and realize I feel old and stiff and should have done something about it years ago when I could. No regrets!—My new motto.

So as I walked, I decided it was the perfect time to visualize myself working out with a personal trainer. I imagined meeting the trainer at the beach, and while I don't know exactly what kind of exercise she would get me to do, I just kept visualizing me working with her. I was running, walking, lifting weights, using one of those big ball things and working up a sweat. I saw myself working hard but at the same time determined to get through it and when I finished my session I felt good. This visualization motivated me to commit myself to call her tomorrow.

For lunch I had tuna salad on a wrap. My afternoon snack was a banana and then some rice crackers. I also drank a cup of tea, and as usual kept up my water intake.

I was really hungry when I arrived home and I was glad I had a couple of those lean frozen meals in the freezer. I chose vegetarian lasagna and I made a salad to go with it. Dessert was one of those single serve ice-creams.

Time for bed.

It's Saturday and so I figure today is the day I should make the phone call to the trainer. The reason I am having so much trouble with making the call is because I know that once I talk to her and agree to meet with her, there is no turning back. No more excuses for not exercising. I can't convince myself that I don't know what to do anymore, because I will have someone to guide me, show me what to do and expect me to work hard at it.

Before I make the call I decide I need to use the visualization exercise again in order to get my motivation back and the confidence it gave me to know I can do this. I recall the vision I used yesterday and go with that. It is a good few minutes spent, because once I am done, I pick up the phone and dial the number. There is no answer, so I leave a message. Well I have done my part and now I can wait for Gabrielle (the trainer) to call me back.

It's raining and I can't go for a walk to the beach. Well I could, but I don't want to, I feel it wouldn't be much fun walking along the beach, in the rain, getting wet. Besides, it's not one of those warm rainy days. It is quite a cold day even though it is the beginning of summer. I decided I would just get in the car and drive to the Mall so I could do some window shopping. I figure walking around the shops could be considered being active.

I get to the shopping centre and regret it instantly because I forget it is only about three weeks until Christmas and already the crowds have swarmed in. I guess it doesn't help that it is raining, which makes it the perfect opportunity to go Christmas shopping instead of hanging out at the beach or doing some outdoor activity.

I wander around for about an hour and a half and decide that is enough bumping into and side stepping around people, so it is time for me to leave. On the way home I vow that next year I will shop online for presents, and wish that I had of thought of it earlier for this year.

I got home, ate lunch and thought about some of the information Crystal had given me when I first went to see her. I remembered that cleaning was a great way to get active—perfect! First I did some vacuuming, which is great, because the townhouse is multiple split levels, and I have a lot of stairs therefore, it takes me a while. I have two bathrooms to clean and I mop the floor in both, as well as the kitchen and laundry. I washed a couple of loads of clothes and hung them on a clothes rack out on the balcony and instead of placing all the clothes into a basket and taking them in one go, I took a few items of clothing at a time which meant walking to the machine, then back to the balcony—it took me about half an hour just to hang my clothes.

Just as I sit down for a rest, my phone rings. "Hi is that Ruby?" "Yes" I answer. "It's Gabby the personal trainer, I am returning your call" "Thanks for calling back" I say, and then continue, explaining to her my reason for calling. We make an appointment for her to come to my place on Monday night. I am still a little unsure about this but I can also feel some excitement creeping in.

It is a great night to stay in make a home-made vegetarian pizza and watch a movie.

Sunday 9pm

Dear HJ,

This morning I had scrambled eggs, grilled tomatoes and mushrooms with one slice of wholemeal toast. I did my cleaning yesterday instead of today so I was unsure of what to do. It is still drizzling, so I thought I would be proactive and just get out there and go for a walk. The weather today was a little warmer, so it wasn't too bad. In fact it was a good thing because I walked to the beach quicker than ever before, I grabbed a coffee on the way home and was sitting on my couch reading the paper and sipping my coffee in no time. All up I was gone for an hour and fifteen minutes, so I was probably walking for about one hour which I am pretty happy with.

After shopping yesterday and reading the paper today, I was becoming aware of just how close we are getting to Christmas. I started to think about the big day or days for that matter because I always get invited to more than one thing and I was feeling the beginnings of a panic attack setting in.

Every Christmas I put on the standard three kilos and struggle for a few months just to get rid of that weight. Some of those kilos have never left my side, hips or tummy. The point is I was stressing out about it. The turkey, the ham, roast vegetables, gravy, sauces, dessert, pretzels, chocolate, the list goes on and on. And it's not just at one person's house, every Christmas event has a mountain of food. I was beginning to think I should have booked myself on a holiday to escape the festivities and feasting that accompanies it.

I calmed myself down and realized I was just being silly and dramatic. I became aware that I was falling into that old trap of thinking of my healthy eating as a diet. If I am eating right and not on a diet, then why am I panicking about Christmas? This time of the year is about spending time with loved ones and enjoying every minute of it. I am a healthy beautiful woman. I am allowed to eat anything I want. Just be sensible, and go with what my body feels the need to have. Don't go overboard and all will be fine. Have fun and enjoy!

Monday 10pm

Dear HJ,

I had a good day today. Breakfast was the usual fruit with Greek yogurt and wheat free muesli. I somehow skipped morning tea (not on purpose) it just didn't happen, but I did get to have a coffee (someone bought it to me). I am grateful for the decent breakfast I eat otherwise I would not have survived. Well, I am sure I would have but it is really unusual for me to skip a meal or snack.

For lunch I ate a tuna salad sandwich and went for a walk which was about 45min duration. I want to be able to tell Gabrielle tonight that I do regular activity. It was very busy at work today with me having to get reports to other floors. Since I started seeing Crystal and following my healthy lifestyle I have been taking the stairs at work instead of using the elevator. I did a lot of that today so I got in more activity than usual.

My afternoon tea consisted of a peach, a cheese stick and a handful of nuts.

Gabrielle was coming over to my place around 7.30pm, so I bought a cooked chicken from the supermarket and ate some of the breast with a salad.

Gabby arrived promptly at 7.30pm and the appointment lasted about an hour. My first impressions of my personal trainer were completely different to my imaginary version of her. I expected her to show up in skin tight lycra leggings, a sports crop top (exposing her well defined six pack), hair in a ponytail and to give me that look that says, "another lazy big assed woman that can't be bothered to look after herself." Well .... I was so wrong. And I prove to myself once again, that I have to stop the way I think in terms of other people. I am always self-conscious of what they think about me and my weight, and yet here I am constantly judging women, in particular, by their looks. Probably from years of being jealous—I am guessing?

Of course, Gabby has a fabulous figure, and so she should, she obviously works hard for it. She was modestly dressed, wearing loose (but not unflattering) fitted yoga pants that skimmed off her tight nicely rounded butt. A tank top that didn't expose her flat tummy, the only thing I had right was the ponytail. Gabby was lovely and made me feel extremely comfortable and I am sure she wasn't secretly thinking about me being a lazy fat ass.

She asked me questions about my health and medical history, and also why I had decided to give her a call.

I explained to her that I started eating healthy about three to four months ago and that I started slowly walking and had picked up the pace over the course of these months and I now felt it was time to get serious about my fitness. I can feel myself improving, but don't know on my own where to go from here.

She was pleased with my answer. She wanted to make sure I wasn't just looking at losing weight and then fall off the wagon once I had reached that magical number on the scale or in my *dress size. Gabby was impressed with my decision to make this about getting myself moving more and improving my fitness levels and physical strength permanently.*

Gabby went through what she thought would be a good activity plan for me (she likes calling it activity because exercise makes it sound like a chore, activity sounds like fun, I have to agree).

I am happy with her ideas and we agreed to meet nice and early on Wednesday morning for my first session.

After meeting Gabby, I am feeling more excited about my decision to include her in my healthy lifestyle. I am not so sure if I will still feel that way while in the middle of my session on Wednesday....

Gabby left and I decided to have a cup of tea. I was feeling a little hungry and wasn't sure what would go with my tea, so I ended up trying a muesli bar. I bought the packet a week ago and hadn't gotten around to eating one of them yet. They are from one of the weight loss companies that you can buy in the grocery store, it was really nice and the perfect portion size for this time of night.

Time for some sleep now.

CHAPTER 11

I t's Wednesday and I am up nice and early for my first training session. Well, I am awake but I am not actually up yet. I am lying in bed wondering if I can still do this. What was I thinking? I shouldn't have a personal trainer. I am nowhere near fit for something like this. I am not a sporty person, never have been and I am certain I never will be.

I let those negative thoughts in, and sent them packing right out the back door of my mind. Time to do a little visualization exercise—I have a couple of minutes to spare.

I close my eyes, and I see myself getting ready for my session. I meet Gabby at the beach, take in the beautiful scenery and feel the cool crisp morning air. I imagine myself following her instructions and achieving the activities with hard work as well as with ease. I see myself as a strong, capable woman ready to improve my fitness levels and excel at any of the exercises given to me, at all times. At the end of the visualization exercise I imagine myself feeling great physically, as well as mentally—my mind is clear, and ready to take on the rest of the day. I walk away smiling.

I get up, and it is time to get dressed and meet Gabby.

As I pull on my workout gear, I remind myself of how far I have come. I eat healthy and I walk on average an hour a day 4 days a week. Best of all, I feel great! I have already imagined how much better I am going to feel from training with Gabby—and with that thought I leave the comforts of my townhouse.

Arriving at the beach, I spot Gabby straight away. This time she is in her tight running leggings but no crop top yet. We spend an hour doing our activity on the beach. Gabby has bought fit balls and small free weights to use, as well as using the wet hard sand for an easy workout, then the soft dry sand for the much harder activities.

The session finishes, and even though I worked my butt off, it wasn't as bad as I thought it would be. I recall my visions of how I wanted the workout to be and apart from the actual exertion I felt from really doing the activity, it is exactly how I pictured. I am now pumped to continue this three times a week, plus my usual walks. I am very surprised, and most of all proud of myself. I do manage to walk away smiling.

Wednesday 9.30pm

Dear HJ,

Today was the first of my "activity" sessions with Gabby. It was hard, but not as bad as I had expected. When I revealed this to Gabby she told me she is lenient at first so clients aren't tempted to run off and never come back for a session again. She explained it is better to build me up to the tough stuff rather than shock me with it in the first session. I am pleased to hear that, even though I am aware it is going to get harder.

I rushed home to get ready and have breakfast. I ate the fruit salad I had prepared before leaving for my session this morning with some yogurt. I quickly grabbed a coffee before walking into the office, because I didn't have time for one at home.

Phew, what a morning! It went quick and before I knew it, lunch time had arrived. I went to the newsagent as I felt the need to look for a new magazine. I ended up buying a fitness one with all sorts of info on exercise, women looking fit and healthy, some inspiring stories of people changing from couch potato to marathon runner, as well as some great new recipes. I went back to work and read the magazine while eating my tuna salad with rice cakes.

The afternoon sailed by with me being super busy and having a lot of energy. I was feeling really good and knew it was a result of my session with Gabby and it has me looking forward to my next one on Friday.

For afternoon tea I had one of the new muesli bars I had tried the other night, and another coffee (I still can't give up my two coffees a day, and so far haven't felt the need to).

For dinner I had a cup of pasta with a tomato based sauce which had a lot of vegetables in it.

I am feeling physically exhausted which is a nice change because I actually feel like I could just collapse into bed and fall into a blissful sleep. I remember back to before I started my healthy lifestyle. The tiredness I felt back then was more of a lethargic feeling, which also resulted in me feeling like I couldn't focus or concentrate on anything. I am beginning to realize I wasn't tired from a big active day, I was tired from not treating my body right and from all the crap I stuffed into it. Things have definitely changed!

Good night ☺

Friday midnight

Dear HJ,

I was up early this morning for my training session. It's amazing how Gabby knows how to put just a little bit more into it to make the second session harder than my first session, but not so hard that I want to give up. I felt good, and again I am glad I made this decision.

Breakfast once again was a rushed fruit salad and yogurt. I would really like a little more time to actually sit and eat my first meal of the day, just to savour and appreciate it but it's only for the mornings I have my sessions and for now that will have to do.

I had a coffee and half a low fat muffin for morning tea. I was a bit disorganized this morning and didn't bring my own snacks to work. I am saving the other half of the muffin for this afternoon to have with some nuts (which I will buy while out at lunch).

It dawns on me during the course of the morning that our work Christmas party is in one week, so I decide my lunch hour would be a good time to start looking for a dress. I have been so consumed by work and focused on how good I feel physically that I have forgotten that Christmas, and all that comes with it, is approaching fast.

I made the mistake of going into a boutique I have always wanted to venture into but always been too embarrassed to because of my size. I am feeling so good about myself at the moment I decided I would have a look in there just for a bit of a dream really. The sales assistant (who looks like mid 40s) sizes me up and down and then proceeds to enquire as to whether I may have been looking for a Christmas present for a friend or maybe my niece? I let the rudeness of the woman cut me like a knife and my emotions lay shattered right there on the boutique floor. I politely told her I was "just looking" and promptly left.

I decided I didn't even want to look in any of the stores that are "appropriate" for my abundant supply of curves, so I headed to my once favourite chocolate store located on the bottom floor of the building.

I stood there looking and staring at all the yummy gooey brown stuff in attractive boxes and wrapping, wondering which one I am going to buy. All of a sudden I am brought back to earth when the sales assistant recognizes me and greets me by name. "Ruby how are you? I haven't seen you in ages. It must be at least two months, maybe more." OMG, she is taking note of how long it has been since my last visit . . . . to the chocolate store? How often did I go into that store? I am now not sure what is more embarrassing the fact that the sales assistant in the boutique thought I had no right being in her store, or the fact that I am on a first name basis with the lady in the chocolate shop.

I told Jenny (the assistant in the chocolate store) I had been too busy for chocolate, which sound so dumb, but I didn't want to go into the real reason for not needing to visit the store. She commented that I look fabulous and I should continue doing whatever it is I am doing to look this way. I thank her and go back to vacantly staring at all the treats lined up on the shelves along the wall.

It's funny, the first thing I noticed is how expensive these chocolates are and I used to purchase them, often! I could buy a punnet of sweet juicy strawberries for half the price of most of these. I told Jenny I was browsing and getting ideas for Christmas and then walked out of the store.

I went back to work feeling a little deflated. Today I ate my salad roll with grated cheese at my desk. I sat staring and processing all the emotions I experienced during forty five minutes of my lunch hour.

I am frustrated and disappointed in myself for letting the sales assistant in the boutique get to me. I am so sensitive and touchy about my size that I expect people to be rude to me about it and to look down on me because of it. I guess I haven't had much self worth over the years and I have spent a lot of time using negative self talk.

Although I have been finding things I like about myself and I am happy with the way I have been progressing, as well as being extremely proud of myself for committing to my healthy lifestyle, I am becoming increasingly aware of what a long process this is (learning to love me). It's not just about eating healthy and learning to love myself and my body, it is also about getting my self-respect back. I am not even sure if it was there in the first place. Learning to Love and Respect myself, isn't going to happen in such a short amount of time. It's like any other relationship, I need to give it time to grow and blossom. I am getting to know myself all over again.

I also need to stop being so paranoid about what other people think of my external image. The lady in the shop could have genuinely been asking me if I needed help to pick something out for someone else. I don't know what people are thinking. I think I know what they are thinking, I assume, and of course, I always think they are judging me and my weight.

I have been learning to like myself more, which is good—but now it is time to start loving myself.

For afternoon tea I ate rice crackers and tzatziki dip.

I left work and went straight to Michelle's. We had previously arranged a night in at her place. She cooked a lovely vegetable and chicken stir-fry with rice noodles—Yum!

After dinner and over one glass of wine I poured my feelings out to Michelle about my lunch time drama. She listened and I could tell she felt bad for me but was trying to cheer me up. I really just wanted someone to listen to me, rather than me writing it down in my journal (which I have done anyway). She then suggested we go out tomorrow and shop for my Christmas party outfit. I am actually looking forward to a little retail therapy with a friend, it will be nice.

After dinner we indulged in some peppermint cream dark chocolate. I made sure I stuck to three pieces which is really all I can manage of that stuff anyway.

I am looking forward to tomorrow—what girl doesn't love to go shopping with a friend, so I am off to bed.

Saturday 11pm

Dear HJ,

I started the day with a hearty breakfast of two boiled eggs, baby spinach, tomato, mushrooms and a slice of wholegrain toast. It was really good, and kept me going until lunchtime.

I met Michelle at 8.30am for a quick coffee before starting on our dress hunt. We hit the stores and looked at anything and everything. That's the good thing about going with a friend, I always feel I have a little more confidence and if I am in a store that appears to be above me (or too small for me, I should say) in the body department, I can always pretend I am there for my thin friend who is standing right next to me.

We were in a department store and I picked out a few things in the size I thought I was. I love the department stores because no one is breathing down your neck and checking if you require another dress size, or wanting to see how you look. You are left to your own device and if you don't like what you see, you can just put it back on your own or hand it to the assistant manning the fitting rooms.

The first dress I try, I am unsure of. It looks weird on me, but I show Michelle anyway . . . . mainly because she keeps bugging me from outside the fitting room "show me! Do you have it on yet? Even if you don't like it, just show me." So ok, I decide to parade the first dress for her.

"Well no wonder you don't like it" she said to me "it's too big for you!" Now I knew I had lost some weight but I figured I couldn't still be any more than a couple of dresses sizes smaller. For this outfit I ended up being three sizes smaller! So Michelle went off to get the next size down for me, while I stand there still, in disbelief.

In every store we went into, I kept picking up a size too big for me. It was really exciting because my brain was telling me I was one size but my body was showing me that I truly was another. Michelle was ecstatic too, she kept telling me how fantastic I looked (in the right dress of course). There were the ones that weren't so great, but I didn't care because I could see how my body was changing. My confidence and self-worth were getting such a boost! It was just what I needed after yesterday.

We stopped for some lunch and instead of facing the food court dilemma, I suggested a café. I ordered a salad sandwich and a glass of water. I sat there wildly ranting to Michelle how I never expected the clothes to look as good as they did, let alone be fitting into three sizes smaller than what I am used to wearing. I guess I should start taking a look at what is in my closet and an even closer look at what I have been wearing to work. I have become so used to certain suits and ensembles for work that even if something has felt loose I have just used a belt to tighten it because I didn't want to believe I had actually lost weight.

I decided on a dress from one of the major department stores. It was a little pricey but it is worth it because it is very flattering to my body shape, and I feel beautiful in it. It is emerald green and suits my complexion. Fits snugly in all the right places and flows in all the areas where I don't want it to be tight.

Michelle has pushed me a little further and made me book in for my make-up to be done at the beautician, the hair I can handle myself. And luckily I am addicted to buying handbags and shoes because I know I have something in my wardrobe to suit the dress.

I ended up buying a banana from the supermarket to have on the way home because I was so hungry.

Michelle and I came back to my place and we made homemade pizza with chicken and vegetables. My treat tonight was two glasses of wine and a single serve low fat cheesecake from a weight loss brand (products that are sold in the supermarket).

Michelle just left, so it is off to bed for me.

CHAPTER 12

Saturday 9am

Dear HJ,

It is Saturday, and one week from when I last wrote to you. Work has been so hectic I managed to write my food down during the week but didn't get around to writing down any of my feelings, challenges or any other daily happenings. I guess this week I haven't really needed to due to it being so busy and me just carrying on doing what I normally do.

I went to my appointment with Crystal on Thursday night. I told her about my exciting shopping trip and the dress I bought for the Christmas party. She seemed genuinely happy for me and proud of what I have achieved.

I told her of my experience last Friday and she acknowledged that I have come a long way with my thought process and was glad I didn't completely derail myself due to the retail assistant. Even though I let her affect me so much, I was able to get my mind back into a happy and positive place after I processed my emotions, and worked out why I had let that woman affect me.

We had a good chat about where I am at and how I feel about Christmas (which is coming up soon and this is my last appointment before the New Year). I told her I am at peace with the holiday season as I am just going to go by instinct and eat what my body tells me to eat. Crystal appeared to be comfortable with this direction and asked me to take photos of me all dressed up for the Christmas party so I can show them to her when I see her next year.

So, last night was my Christmas party. We had it in a really swish restaurant in the city with magnificent views of the harbour. The food was absolutely beautiful and the wine was the best I have ever tasted (guess I don't spend enough on it).

Everyone looked stunning and I think I scrubbed up pretty well myself. I received a lot of compliments from colleagues both males and females, which was really nice. People that I barely speak to at work were all of a sudden coming up to me and chatting as if we are lifelong friends, this has never happened to me at work events before. Maybe I came across as aloof or shy because of my lack of confidence. Maybe they didn't want to talk to me because I was fat. The latter is my negative version of how I think people view me and because of this, I don't think I have been a very approachable person.

A few of the girls came up to me telling me they are sure I had lost weight. One colleague in particular (Susan) told me that not only had I lost weight, but I was looking radiant. She went on about how clear my eyes are and how wonderful my skin is. Wow! This kind of conversation just urges me on and motivates me to keep up my healthy eating and activity. I do know it is working, but sometimes I need confirmation that proves other people are seeing what I am feeling. A bit of attention from other people never goes astray.

I didn't bother worrying about my food intake and to be honest I don't think I really needed to. Waiters came around with dishes of small portions of meals with quite a variety to choose from and I didn't accept every dish that was on offer. What I ate was enough to keep me satisfied. The desserts were in bite size portions and so after sampling three of the options I felt like I had definitely had enough. The wine kept flowing and in my already buzzing mood, I probably went slightly overboard but the only disappointment I have with myself about that is the fact that I am a little hung over.

All in all it was a fabulous night and I am glad I had fun.
It's sad but true that this is the first Christmas party I have
honestly enjoyed.
I just ate eggs and vegetables for breakfast, and I am now
going for a walk to the beach.
Bye for now.

I walk out the door and I am feeling very pleased with myself. I have kept up my healthy eating lifestyle for five months now, which doesn't sound like much but it's a huge achievement for me. Most programs I began in the past, only lasted two months at the most.

A couple of years ago, I saw a nutritionist and followed her healthy eating plan. I think I stuck to it for about two months. It was similar to what I am doing now, in the sense that it was based on eating healthy foods. The difference was she made up a menu plan for me to follow. Unfortunately I felt quite restricted because none of the foods I enjoy, such as chocolate or chips, were anywhere on my menu plan, not even a fun size version! I was supposed to swap bad foods for good foods. For example, she suggested swapping yummy crispy potato chips for crunchy carrot sticks or chocolate for strawberries . . . . yeah that doesn't really work. The concept was good but it didn't suit me and my needs.

In the end, I didn't lose any weight (which was the whole reason for me going on that plan), because I felt deprived and ended up sneaking junk food in somewhere during the day. I found it difficult to socialize too. There was no allowance for eating out. It was suggested that I ate before going out and then ordering a salad without dressing in a restaurant. I just decided not venture out of the house which ended up in me not having any fun. Thinking back I am surprised I lasted two months but that is probably because I snuck some "naughty" food into my mouth.

After my first meeting with Crystal I was a little skeptical. I thought I knew it all and had tried everything which left me with no hope. Her concept seemed to be like all the other plans out there. What's the difference? It is not a plan, it's a way of life. The moment I got my head around that, is the moment my body and mind clicked together and became in tune with each other to achieve my goal of becoming healthy and fit.

I am loving the whole process of learning about myself—mind and body! I may be a little hung over but it is another fantastic day. Christmas is just around the corner and this time instead of stressing about the fact that I will put on weight, I am excited to spend the day with family and having a good time.

CHAPTER 13

Dear HJ,

It is getting longer between me writing to you. I guess that is a good thing because it means I am not dependent on writing down my thoughts anymore and I am confident in knowing that the majority of the time I am on the right track.

Christmas is done and dusted. The time I spent with my family was really special this year and I think I noticed it more because I felt really relaxed. We all sat back with an abundance of conversation and laughed a lot. I have to say it was the best Christmas as an adult I have had.

I finished work a few days before Christmas and spent that time buying presents and socializing. I wasn't even panicking about the fact that I had left everything to the last minute. The truth is it kept me busy and active.

I was invited to Nat's house for Christmas Eve along with many other friends. It was magical. She decorated her place so beautifully. The table was set with name tags, a lovely centerpiece, matching dinnerware and napkins . . . . I love this time of the year.

We had a great night. There was a lot of food on the table and it dawned on me while I was sitting there how most of us try to eat a large portion of every dish on the table at Christmas. Why? It's not food we can't cook or access any other time of the year. It's a meal just like any other, just with a celebration attached to it. There are some great choices on this table. There is turkey, ham, chicken and vegetables. The vegetables probably have a little more oil or fat to what I am now used to, but I don't need to pile my plate high to enjoy them.

I decided on a sensible portion of turkey, two squares of potato, three pieces of sweet potato and lots of cauliflower and broccoli (they were steamed) and a spoonful of peas and corn. Dessert was a choice of pavlova or Christmas pudding. I decided on a small piece of pavlova, it was loaded with fruit and so I decided to eat the fruit first and then if I needed to, I could eat the meringue and I left the cream until last. Some of the meringue and the cream were left (which was a first for me).

Danni was watching me the whole time. It was a little unnerving. And at the moment the conversation switched to me with everyone remarking how I am looking healthy and slim was nice, and great for my ego, but I was sure I could feel her eyes stinging me even more. I am not shy of receiving positive attention and compliments but it is difficult when it feels like someone is not on the same page as everyone else. I just have to accept that she may be feeling a little jealous and let it go, I can't do anything about it, only Danni can, and only if she wants to.

We finished the festive eating for the evening and were all kicking back with a few drinks. Conversations broke off into little sections of the room, and it was then that Danni approached me. She admitted to me that she had been feeling resentful towards me because every time she saw me, I was shrinking more and more in size. Danni opened up to me about how at one stage she was worried she would be the only large sized girl in our group. I was taken aback by this admission while at the same time reminding myself of how immature she can be. She then went on to say how she had a real good look at herself and realized she needed to stop bringing everyone else down with her, she is now aware that in order to change what she is not happy about, she has to change the way she thinks.

Our conversation was very eye opening. We talked for what seemed like hours. Danni told me that in the end instead of *seeing me as the shrinking enemy because we weren't on the same "let's be fat girls' together" level anymore, she began to see me as inspiration and she was actually observing me for some motivation. Interesting . . . . I didn't realize staring at me could be motivating, but if it worked for her then so be it.*

We finished off our conversation with me giving her Crystal's number, and her promising that instead of seeing this week as her long last feasting supper, she will be trying to cut down her portion sizes and make healthier choices. I reassured her that she was on the right track.

I hope Danni is truly ready and she does as well I am doing. Everyone deserves to be happy, healthy and fit.

So HJ, the next day of course was Christmas.

I arrived early at my parents place so I could help prepare the food. Emmy and Jeff were there too and we kicked off the morning with opening gifts and eating (of course). My mum's idea of breakfast is chocolate coated sultanas and peanuts with pretzels. I knew I was going to feel like crap before the day had even begun so I suggested we at least cook some eggs and toast for us all to eat before starting on the sugar and salt.

Everyone looked relieved at my idea but I think mum was a little put out. Apparently it is tradition to start Christmas day on as little nutritious food as possible. Yes, I do remember using Christmas in previous years as an excuse to binge on junk food all day long. We have plenty of hours left in the day to feast on the large amounts of goodies my mum has purchased but let's at least do it on a satisfied stomach.

We ate our hearty breakfast and in the end I think mum agreed it was "sensible" because as tradition would have it, she opened a bottle of champagne. Mum admitted that without the eggs and toast she would have been a giggling mess already.

Preparations for dinner began and the day was moving along very fast. I did end up indulging in the sultanas, nuts and pretzels, not to mention the crackers, cheese and dip that was on offer for lunch. I was enjoying the binge at the time. By the way I also decided I wasn't going to worry about my visualization tools for Christmas day, I just wanted to see how I would go on my own.

By 3.30pm the house was full with aunts, uncles, cousins and one set of grandparents. An uncle of mine walked in the door and decided to announce very loudly "Geez, Ruby you've lost a lot of chub haven't you. Now your ass can find the dining chair!" Oh my god! How embarrassing!! Let's face, the man has never been known to have any tact, but that was just down—right rude. I just laughed it off. Even though his comment was offensive and embarrassing, I guess I can see the compliment in there somewhere.

One of my aunt's came up and displayed her disgust with his behaviour and gently acknowledged to me how wonderful she thought I looked. "You have lost weight dear" she said "and you look really healthy and happy!" A couple of cousins sitting in ear shot enthusiastically agreed which was lovely. They all wanted to know what finally worked for me. I told them I was just being sensible and following a healthy lifestyle. I also mentioned how I had started walking and then moved on to working with a personal trainer. There were "oohs" and "ahs" echoing the room. I think I got a little shy with all the attention but at the same time I loved it. Usually it's my sister that receives the compliments not me.

Christmas dinner was beautiful. I loved the conversation that consisted of current world events, what's happening with everyone's jobs, who's having babies, couples that have announced their engagements as well as some walks down memory lane. By the end of the night, ninety-five percent of my family were unbuttoning their pants or wishing they had worn a more forgiving dress and cursing that the amount of food they had consumed will stick to their thighs for the next year.

I know I did over do it myself on Christmas day, I felt lethargic, my mouth was really dry (probably from all that sugar and salt) and in general I didn't feel as good as I normally do. For a few seconds I felt guilty and disappointed in myself for going to the extreme with the food but quickly got over it because I will never be perfect when it comes to healthy eating and I don't need to be. For the majority of the time I pack a lot of vitamins and minerals into my body through the foods I choose to eat. Christmas is one day and maybe next year I will remember how I felt at 10pm that night and remind myself not to make the same mistake, but then again, it is Christmas, so we will just have to wait and see.

I reminded myself tomorrow is a brand new day to start all over again and that is what I did.

Boxing day, we were invited to spend the day with other family that couldn't make it to my parents' house for Christmas. Once again when I walked through the door cousins were commenting on my weight loss and the fact that I look healthy. "You are looking so fit Ruby" someone said to me. Fit! Wow the word "fit" and "Ruby," have never been in the same sentence together before—ever. Imagine what I will look like when I have been going to my activity sessions for a few months. This comment was a huge boost and I found I was back on track with the healthy food for the whole day. I have to admit that on this occasion there was a lot of fruit and salad on offer. I think everyone needed it after yesterday.

Today is the day after Boxing Day and I am relieved to be spending the day at home, alone. I received a lot of gift cards over Christmas, so I decided it is time to throw some of the large clothes in my wardrobe out. A part of me was worried about getting rid of my larger clothes in case I need them again, but then I realized how ridiculous this was, because I will remain healthy and I won't be putting on weight again. I also need to remind myself to live in the present, and right now I am in need of some clothes, that fit, so I am going to have fun shopping for them.

Okay HJ time for me to attack my closet. Talk to you soon.

New Years Day 10pm

Dear HJ,

It has once again been a few days since I last wrote. Crystal did mention to me that when I find I am not writing my journal *as much, it is a sign that I am just living a healthy lifestyle, it has become a habit and is now the way I live. I definitely see this as positive. I have finally come to a point in my life where I am less likely to have negative thoughts about my appearance, my body, and anything to do with my image. My paranoia of how I think people view me has also subsided, as I am less likely to make up a scenario in my head of what a person is thinking of me.*

The last time I wrote I was about to go through my wardrobe. I did and it was freeing. I threw out so many clothes. I packed up many boxes, and then took them to a charity bin and I like to think someone somewhere can use them.

The next day I took myself shopping and purchased some lovely clothes. I still have issues taking the size too big for me into the fitting room, but I am learning to automatically go down to the next size. I am generally a size 16 at the moment and I can feel a lot of them are slightly loose. There are quite a few 16's in my closet (previous years of wishful thinking) and so I got game and bought a few of the larger 14's and I am confident this isn't a mistake.

It was New Year's Eve yesterday, and I was invited to a friend's place for a party. I had a great time chatting, dancing and seeing the New Year in with a bunch of great people. Danni was there, and even though it had only been a week since I had last seen her, she looked different—happier. She excitedly told me about how she had been following a healthy lifestyle and she was extremely proud of herself for managing to keep it up over Christmas. She also mentioned she had rung Crystal during the week enquiring about an appointment. Crystal didn't answer the call (probably because of Christmas) but she did however, send her a text with a couple of choices for appointment bookings. Danni is over the moon that she is booked in to see her next week.

This is a special new year for me because for the first time ever, I have not made a resolution that consists of going on a diet, losing weight, no sugar for the year, no bread for the year or a juice diet for the first month etc, and then going through the disappointment of not following through with it. I am healthy, I am (becoming) fit and the bonus is I have lost weight along the way. In fact, the weight is not lost, because when something is lost there is the possibility of finding it again. Instead I would like to say I reduced my body size and shape. Crystal is going to love that!

No more New Year's Resolutions for me.

Time for me to go do some activity. Bye for now.

CHAPTER 14

I started my healthy lifestyle appointments with Crystal six months ago, and today, will be my last one before I go on to monthly appointments with her. I can't believe how quickly the time has gone. Probably three months into my lifestyle change, I didn't think the time was flying, but now that I have made it to six months, I can really say it has sailed by.

I am in Crystal's waiting room and I feel like I belong because I have been visiting this place for six months. I sit patiently while she finishes up with her previous client. As Crystal and her client leave the room I look in their direction as one does. I smile and quickly look away because the lady looks like she has only just started coming here and I don't want her to feel self conscious by appearing to be staring at her. I briefly reflect how I felt the first day I entered this office. Although I felt a small amount of excitement of a journey that lay ahead of me, I also felt daunted by not knowing what was on the path I was about to take.

"Hi Ruby, come on in." We both sit in the comfortable chairs provided. "Can you believe it has been six months since your first appointment?" says Crystal. "No" I say, a little coy and childishly, although I am not sure why?

"I have seen a lot of changes within you both inside and out" she smiles. "Along the way we have discussed in depth your successes, worries, fears and challenges. So I do know what you have been feeling while travelling down this path but I would like to hear today, how you are feeling in the present moment."

"I feel great!" I say. I feel the need to elaborate so I go on, "I feel extremely healthy, energetic and light." Crystal smiles and asks me to explain what I mean by "light." "Well when I walk, I feel like I am floating. I know I have lost weight so I guess I'm not carrying any excess baggage anymore." Crystal laughs, "That's a positive."

"And when you say 'healthy,' how is it different from before? I mean you weren't really unhealthy when you started your new lifestyle, so can you explain to me what is different?"

"Yes, I don't feel lethargic like I used to. My energy levels have increased from not consuming too many high in sugar/ high in fat foods, as well as from the activity I am doing. I sleep better at night. I think clearer during the day and feel like I have better focus when doing a task which means I can finish it well, and move on to the next task. I also noticed I haven't been sick since starting my healthy lifestyle. I have been around family and friends when they have had colds and I didn't get one at all."

"That's great Ruby! You will also find that if you do happen to get sick, you will get over it quicker because you are healthier and fitter."

"So Ruby now that you have been coming to see me for six months, and you are settled in your healthy lifestyle, would you like to know how much weight you have lost?"

Even though my new and improved lifestyle was all about my getting healthy and fit, I am curious and excited to find out how much weight I have lost. Because remember, this is the bonus of changing the way I thought about myself, my body and my eating habits. "Yes" I answer.

"Ruby you have reduced your weight by twenty two kilos." "Really? No, I couldn't . . . . is that really possible?" Crystal was smiling a nodding her head. "Did you think it would be that much Ruby?" "It was obvious to me I had lost a bit of weight because I have dropped quite a few dress sizes, it just didn't dawn on me it would be that much. I became so focused on feeling healthy that I just forgot about any numbers to do with weight."

It was an honest answer, and because I wasn't being weighed in at every session, I really didn't have any numbers to focus on at all. I didn't have to watch my weight go up on the scales or stay the same, only to be disappointed because I knew how hard I had worked, and yet the scales didn't prove it with the results I would have been expecting. My goal became my health and fitness, not a number on the scales or my dress size, therefore, the hard work I was putting in was not to see any numbers change, but to feel the change physically.

I was so happy I wanted to jump up and hug Crystal.

"Ruby, I am more than confident that you can continue with your healthy lifestyle on your own and I look forward to seeing you in a month's time, just to catch up on where you are at. If you ever need to talk about anything, you can call me, but somehow I don't think you will need to." She says with such pride in her eyes, and I smile proudly back.

I walk away with my head held high because I have already achieved more than I thought I ever could and I am looking forward to continuing and furthering my success in getting fitter and healthier.

CHAPTER 15

The last six months have flown by. I have continued with my lifestyle as normal, it just second nature for me to eat the way I do, and include activity at least three times a week. I have kept up my visits with Crystal every month for the last five months, which have continued to be insightful, motivational and an opportunity for me to learn more every time I sit in her office. Today is my last session with Crystal, which marks the twelve month anniversary from when I began my healthy eating path.

I deliberately arrive early so I can sit in the waiting room to gather fifteen minutes of thoughts and reflection. I feel so far removed physically and mentally from where I was when I first ventured into this office twelve months ago.

The transition I have made, from a shy, unhappy, large well dressed woman, who struggled to breathe while walking up a flight of stairs, to a confident, healthy, strong, fit and happy well dressed young woman who can now run up several flights of stairs, hasn't been smooth sailing. I couldn't have done it, without changing a lot of my inner speech that would normally create walls and blockages. I chipped at those obstacles that I had created over the years and finally knocked them all to the ground with a sledge hammer.

Eventually I found "Ruby"—the real Ruby, who was hiding in the middle of a great big comfortable sack of wool. The layers started to peel off when I realized I needed to be kind to myself, with no more negative self talk, no more name calling, and no more self sabotage.

I discovered the "no more diet" option. By eating naturally with healthy and nutritious foods that replenish my body and soul, I felt whole. I became aware that when I had previously dieted, I felt as though I was punishing myself for being fat. I had to deprive or restrict myself of the foods that were known as rewards or treats. And because I had to diet, I saw myself unworthy of being a normal person. In my mind, I could never see myself as the type of person that didn't need to diet, the person that wasn't fat and didn't eat the wrong foods. I was always fat Ruby.

Eventually, I told myself I was worthy of being a normal person that didn't need to diet. I was beautiful and I deserved to be happy and healthy. Instead of seeing myself as thin, I visualized a healthy, fit and strong independent woman, who could take on the world.

My healthy eating path stayed strong because I didn't have any limitations or restrictions and I didn't deprive myself. There was no lack of motivation because I wasn't obsessed with numbers on a scale and numbers lost each week on that scale. I didn't have a "plateau" because I had no idea of what my weight was, therefore, I was unaware if it happened to stabilize for a week or two.

I enjoyed my life before, but I feel as though I enjoy it even more now. I am really happy but it's not just because I eat healthy and have lost weight, it is also because of the fact that I am quite active and I have that get up and go that I didn't experience before. The less energy I had, the less motivation I felt to do anything. My social life has improved, I actually feel like going out and having fun. I talk to more people at work and I even want to see family more often.

I love life and I feel I have so much to give which is why I quit my job as a PA and Paralegal. I woke up one day and realized that the career I was in, did not serve my purpose in life. I would never have had the courage to give up my well paid employment if I hadn't embarked on a lifestyle change. The last twelve months has been a huge journey of self discovery in many ways, and I want to make sure I devote the rest of my life doing something every day that I enjoy.

I am about to begin a new journey—one of study. I have chosen psychology (for various reasons). One day I would like to be able to help people with their body, their food habits, the way they treat themselves, and help them look into themselves deeper and discover more about how to connect their body and their mind. I would like to help clients explore why they eat the way they do, and why they struggle with their weight. I am really looking forward to my new career path.

My thoughts are broken by Crystal appearing and inviting me into her office. "So Ruby, here we are—one year since we first met, and this is your last appointment with me." I nearly cry. I have become slightly attached to Crystal, but there is no reason for me to visit anymore. I am where I need to be in my life. I naturally eat well—I don't even have to think about it anymore. I exercise and actually enjoy it! It is time to open a space for someone else who needs Crystal's guidance.

I excitedly told Crystal about my new adventure, she was extremely happy for me. "You will be very successful in your new role Ruby as a student and then as a psychologist and I wish you all the best. I am sure we can team up some time. You may be able to help me with any clients that need that little extra help and attention".

"So for one last time in this office would you like to know how much weight you have removed over this last year?" Yes, I am very keen, so I nod to Crystal. "Ruby you have gone down 36.5 kilos! That was an average of 700 grams a week which is fantastic. You are in a healthy weight range for your height and your measurements are amazing with you getting rid of a lot of inches everywhere."

"Yippee!" I knew I had gone down a lot in my weight because I am now a size 10. The number on the scales aren't really important to me because I am fit and toned everywhere which is so surreal to me, and although I spent many days imagining it to be real, I never physically felt it or saw it, until now. I have to admit, for the first time ever I am extremely pleased when I see my reflection in the mirror.

"Well Ruby, I have enjoyed coaching you. It is now forever up to you to continue coaching yourself."

I gave Crystal a hug, we then said our goodbyes and I headed out to meet some friends at the mall.

No more food or emotional journaling for me. I am off to live my life like any other healthy young twenty seven year old.

A few days after my last visit to Crystal I received a letter from her in the mail. It reads;

Dear Ruby,

Congratulations!

I am so happy you achieved your goal of becoming healthy and fit. I know you will find it easy to maintain, because you have truly made the transition from old negative habits, to a new positive view on yourself and life. During this process your intuition and awareness of what your body needs has been fine tuned and I am confident it will now stay with you for life.

During our sessions, as I do with any other client, I always made sure that the time was utilised for you and anything you wished to question or talk about. I feel we touched some pretty challenging issues that you have faced your whole life and I am confident you have worked through them enough in order to deal with them should they pop up again at any time in the future.

When any client of mine graduates from their sessions with me I always send them a letter congratulating them of their personal success as well as my background and what made me become a healthy lifestyle coach.

I, like many of my clients struggled with my weight from the time I was a young child. Other kids at school teased me for being overweight, as did some of my family members—much like you experienced.

By the time I reached high school I was still overweight and within two years of being there I had put on more weight. I wasn't heavily obese, but it was enough to draw attention from the so called "perfect" bullies who felt they had the right to call me fat, ugly cow or elephant—and the list goes on. I made other friends just like me and they became my security blanket.

When I was sixteen, I left school and attended a drama course for about a year. This ended up being a great choice for me, as I was finally in a class of people that didn't seem to care what I looked like. I was the youngest and so I guess a lot of the students took on a big brother or sister role with me. Most of them were in their 20s, 30s and a couple of them even in their 40s. My confidence began to grow because I wasn't constantly being told I was ugly or fat.

While attending the course I gained some knowledge of how to take care of myself. For example we were encouraged not to eat big meals, or junk food before movement and dance classes. I found I was losing weight and feeling healthier. I became more aware of my body and how to treat it.

I decided to go back to school the next year and complete my last two years. This time I was in a different grade with students I didn't know and for some reason I didn't experience any teasing . . . . I think it's because I was thinner when I went back to school—amazing hey!

I gained a boyfriend and managed to keep my weight down. I never felt good enough for him because he made it quite clear he was used to being with girls more "glamorous" than me. It also didn't help that he never really gave out compliments, and he never made me feel beautiful. Although later down the track, I realized it's not up to someone else to make you feel beautiful, it is up to you to see your own beauty, and that, I did.

My weight fluctuated throughout my early twenties, I spent many years worrying about and consumed by my weight. "Do I look thin enough?" "Is my body good enough to wear this dress?" "Am I attractive enough?" I don't need to keep going, because you know how the self talk goes.

I lost my boyfriend (which wasn't a bad thing), started enjoying my time with girlfriends which meant dining out, cooking up a storm at home once a week with each other, lots of food to nibble on before we went out, or cooked dinner. Before I knew it, my skirts were getting tighter and dresses busting at the seams.

I met my husband and at the same time started a new role in a weight loss company as a consultant trying to help other people lose weight. My husband and I spent two years going to restaurants for lunch and dinner, as well as going out with friends and enjoying a lot of barbeques. The weight was packing on, quite quickly, and I found myself buying the next one and then two sizes up whenever I needed clothes.

The year leading up to our wedding was the perfect opportunity and motivation for me to get my weight down and back to normal, but we socialized so much and it seemed food was more important to me than being thin for the wedding, so when the big day arrived, I hadn't lost much weight at all. I was slightly disappointed about this, but I also realized my weight was the least important thing about my wedding day.

I thought working in a weight loss company would have been my answer . . . . but it wasn't. There was nothing wrong with their program, I just wasn't ready. It was a diet to me—something that was supposed to get me from fat, to skinny. Each time I tried a diet, whether it was one from a magazine or the one I promoted in my job, I failed.

I spent many years being unhappy with my weight, going up and down like a yo-yo. I bought magazines with all the latest fad diets and I bought all the foods I needed to follow the diets properly . . . . but I never did. I hated photos of myself, I didn't like the clothes I was wearing but, worst of all I never felt healthy. And, I didn't look healthy.

I began to realize that I had put so much emphasis on the fact that I looked overweight and not being able to wear the right clothes, I lost perspective on where I really needed to be with my body, healthy, fit and feeling good.

Instead of buying magazines with fad diets, I started reading the ones with inspirational stories of real people that took charge of their life and their health. I noticed a pattern forming around the successful weight loss stories within the magazines—they all reduced their size because they were ready to be healthy and fit. Their first priority was being healthy for themselves which then goes down the line to being there for their children, spouses, grandchildren and family in general. They all wanted to keep up with life, to live it and enjoy it.

I decided that's what I wanted too. I needed to be healthy and feel fit. At this point I had quit my role as a Weight Loss

Consultant, it didn't serve a purpose with me anymore, but it gave me the foundations I needed for my next step. I focused on getting myself to where I wanted to be physically and mentally, and then eventually leading me to where I am today and I am forever grateful for that.

I started a food journal. For me, I found counting calories was the way to go. It meant I could still have any of the foods I enjoyed while at the same time learning about portion sizes and nutritional values of various foods.

Walking was my only form of exercise. At first my husband joined me showing his support for what I was doing. Then a friend of mine showed her interest in wanting to exercise which made it a fun hour of walking and chatting.

Within weeks, I was feeling better and within months I felt healthier and I was much happier. Just like you, I found I was less tired, more energized, didn't pick up illnesses as quickly and could finally walk up a hill without feeling like I was carrying a sack of potatoes.

My weight dropped which of course is the added bonus and I was ecstatic about that. I got to a certain point with my weight and stayed there for quite a few years. I didn't mind because I was healthy and active.

This is when I decided I wanted to coach people in leading a healthy lifestyle and I have been doing it for a few years now—I love it! I lost weight and became healthy by still enjoying a variety of food. I get annoyed when I hear people say they are omitting certain food groups with the aim of losing weight. I still ate bread, past, rice and potatoes, as well as dairy and the occasional treat, why can they? I decided it was time to show people that they don't have to go without, in order to have a healthy body.

Even though it is my job, I too can be susceptible to set backs and falling into old bad habits, which is what happened about two years ago.

I became aware that I was back to giving myself a serve of pasta that would feed four people. I was doing the same thing with rice, possibly more. I always made sure I had chocolate in the house so I could consume it every day, as well as eating ice-cream every night. I kept thinking I could get away with it because I was at a healthy weight and I managed to maintain it for quite a few years.

After a few months of doing this though, I became aware I wasn't feeling as healthy as what I had been. I knew I was going overboard with a lot of things. This reminded me that it wasn't about my weight and stabilizing the number on the scales or my dress size it was all about how I felt physically. Even though my weight was in a healthy range, nothing else was. Lacking in energy and picking up illnesses again, I knew it was time to stop. I quit buying ice-cream altogether. I cut down the chocolate, with the occasional dark chocolate instead and I went back to measuring pasta and rice. This time, it didn't take long for me to get back to feeling great again.

I made a couple of other changes. For example instead of a sandwich for lunch I began eating cottage cheese with salad (I include a huge amount of lettuce, it barely fits in the bowl), yogurt and fruit or eggs for breakfast and dinner is mainly vegetables (potatoes included) with a bean mix or some other protein that isn't meat (I am vegetarian by the way). It works for me and I feel better than I ever have.

I spent many years listening to my body in order to find out what works for it and what doesn't. I take the time to stop and feel what is going on inside of me once I have eaten certain foods. Do I feel heavy after eating that? Do I feel energized or tired from eating that? Am I jittery from too much sugar or caffeine? It's amazing what our bodies can tell us if we just take the time to listen. I also discovered that little click in my brain that tells me where to stop on that family sized chocolate block that I occasionally decide to buy and munch on.

I love and respect myself. I didn't always. I realized that in order for me to be love and respected by other people, I have to be able to feel it for myself first. I became aware that I needed to treat my body better, it is the only one I have. Each day I tell myself I am grateful for the healthy and strong body I live in.

I am responsible for feeding this body healthy fuel, keeping it active and treating it with respect. And that is what I choose to do, every day.

During the course of this last year Ruby, I have seen you change from a girl who didn't have a lot of self-worth or respect, to a woman who learnt to love herself, respect the person she is, the body she lives in and transform into a healthy, fit, strong being.

You should be extremely proud of yourself. I may have been your coach to guide you and listen to your positive and negative experiences or thoughts, but you take full credit for achieving the goal you set out to achieve. You did it all. You made decisions you never thought you would make and took on challenges you didn't think you were capable of getting through, but you did. Now it is time to live the rest of your life as the person you have always wanted to be.

I wish you all the best with your studies—I know you will be a star pupil.

Good bye for now Ruby, I am sure we will cross paths in the future.

Love Crystal.

Reading Crystal's letter has brought me to tears. Hearing how she came to be a Healthy Lifestyle Coach and struggled in her life with her weight, and had experiences in her life similar to my own, has made me realize just how much she could relate to my story. I understand now where her empathy and compassion toward her clients comes from.

I am also crying for the Ruby I once knew, who struggled with her body image, who was teased as a child for being fat, who felt like she was being judged all the time because she was fat, who had little self-respect for herself and who never knew how to change in order to get to where she wanted.

I also have happy tears for the Ruby I am getting to know, who loves herself, who is strong, who believes she is beautiful, who doesn't care what other people think anymore, and who finally found a way to change how she feels and treats herself in order to get to where she belongs.

Right now, I am where I want to be in this present moment, and I know for sure that I will continue my path of belonging, by making the most of each day and living it, right here and now. Not in my mind, not in the past and not in the future. Right now, I belong to today, and today I feel like the most beautiful human being in the world.

I have thanked Crystal for supporting me as my healthy lifestyle coach, for guiding me when I needed to be led, and for listening to me when I needed to be heard. I am forever grateful that she has starred in my life.

Most of all, I have thanked Ruby. I am happy and confident that I will never have to say "Diet starts tomorrow," ever again.

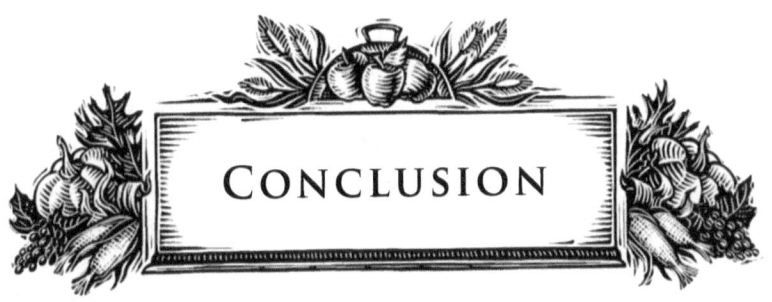

CONCLUSION

Let's take a look at some of the hints and tips Ruby followed;

- Use a journal. Even though you are not dieting, a journal is a good way to keep track of the foods you eat. It gives you an indication of what works for you and what doesn't, as well as the opportunity to see how often you may have included not so healthy foods.
- By looking back through your journal, you can then see where you may be able to improve your healthy eating, or where you may have missed things and realize why you were so hungry, as well as where you can find alternatives for the foods you really love, but may not be your best options.
- Use your journal to record how you are feeling, about anything. Write down any emotions you have whilst progressing on your healthy path, as well as any challenges, negativity from yourself or others, the positives, the discoveries, and any affirmations you use to get you motivated and the ones that keep you going forward. A journal to record your feelings and emotions will give you an indication of where you need to work most on yourself, as well as having those light bulb moments as to why you may feel or react a certain way towards a variety of situations or challenges in your life when it comes to your diet, your health and your body.

- Look at your portion sizes. Most of us have grown accustomed to large meals, for every meal of the day. We cook a lot and we hate to waste food. If this is one of your dilemmas then I suggest using a measuring cup, especially for foods such as pasta, rice and noodles. Even if the food you are eating is healthy, you still need to watch the portion size. For example, a potato is good for you. It has vitamins in it that your body needs, but it is better for you to eat one, than three. The same goes for most foods, but you can definitely bulk up on that garden salad that consists of lettuce, tomato and cucumber. There are many other vegetables you can eat a lot of, so go ahead and do some research.

- If you are unsure of what a portion size of something is, then check out the table on the packet. The table informs you of the weight for one serve, or how many pieces are one serve etc. You could also check with a professional such as a nutritionist, there are also examples on websites, or you could just go with a small plate and bowl, which is a good start. Some even suggest using smaller forks and spoons.

- Change any negative self talk to positive thoughts. For example, don't call yourself lazy, fat, a pig or anything else that has negative words toward your weight or body or yourself in general. No feelings of guilt are allowed either. If you eat something you feel isn't beneficial to your health and wellbeing, then just accept what you have done, and move on, don't dwell on it.

- Start loving yourself and having respect for who you are. Tell yourself you are beautiful, healthy, strong and capable of leading a life full of energy and motivation. You could say things to yourself such as: "Reaching optimum health is important to me." "I am filling my body with healthy nutritious foods." "90% of the food I put into my body will be nutritious and beneficial to my body." "I can eat whatever I want, so I choose foods that are nutritious."

- Take time out of the equation. There are no time limits for a healthy lifestyle. When we go on "diets" we follow them for a certain amount of weeks, or months. So we tend to focus on the time we will be on the diet, giving us a deadline for when we will be at our skinny goal. This is another restriction, and kind of like a deprivation as we are focused on reaching that deadline to lose pounds and have the body we always dreamed of. We become impatient with this "time" and set ourselves up for disappointment if we don't get to our goal by the end of it.

- It's amazing too, how many of us will stick to the time frame set out, maybe even reach our goal, and then "woo hoo" it's back to old habits once again, because we served our time on a diet and we are back to having our freedom.

- By accepting that you are living a healthy lifestyle, then the only goal you have is to eat and remain healthy. This means, there are no time limits, as it should be a way of life forever. What a fantastic way to be for the rest of your life.

- Be kind to yourself. Most of us find it easier to be kind to other people over ourselves. It's not possible to be positive 100% of the time, so if you have a negative thought about yourself or are feeling disappointed about something you have done, think it, feel it, and then let it pass. Drop it as quickly as possible and then go on with a positive thought or action.

- You are not on a diet. There is no more dieting. Make a commitment to your body and soul to start a healthy lifestyle, and maintain the healthy path. There is no more losing weight. If you lose ten kilos do you really want to find it again? I didn't think so. Instead, look at it as reducing your weight or dropping a size or two. But remember, the focus isn't your weight it is about improving your health.

- Just because you choose to follow a healthy lifestyle doesn't mean you can't go out. If you are going to a café or restaurant for a meal, see if they have a website and check out their menu previous to arriving at the venue. This will give you an idea of what will be the best option for you to order. Once you have made your mind up about what you are going to eat, you are less likely to change it later on.

- If you have been invited to a dinner party at someone's house, then just go with what is on offer. You can't control what you eat one-hundred percent of the time. There will be occasions where the best option is the only option that is available to you at the time. The aim is to eat healthy, the majority of the time, therefore, you need to allow for eating out and having fun, without the guilt.

- Following a healthy lifestyle also means there is no deprivation. If you feel like eating a chocolate bar, then you can eat one. If you have a craving for chips then go ahead and have them. Always take the time first to stop and ask yourself why you feel the need to eat something unhealthy. Is it emotional? Is it from stress? Are you after something sweet, and if so can this be satisfied with a piece of fruit? Do you want the taste of something savoury, or is it the crunch you are after? Are you bored or hungry? If you are hungry, will this choice of food actually be substantial enough to sustain your hunger?

- Other questions to ask; "is this beneficial to my healthy lifestyle?" "How will eating this be beneficial to my body that thrives on vitamins and minerals?" "I might feel good while eating this, but how will I feel once I have eaten this?"

- If you choose to eat something that is not healthy or nutritious, then it is important to not feel guilty after consuming it. Eat it, enjoy it, and then move on with your day as normal. Don't fall into the trap of thinking you have ruined your day of healthy eating, and therefore, it is easier to continue down the path of feasting on junk food for the rest of the day. Accept that the craving you had is over and done. It's not a craving or a treat if you do it every day or more than once a day so try to keep them to a minimum.

- Listen to your body. After eating a large meal, or a meal that doesn't have much nutritional value in it take note of how you feel. Don't think about the taste or how you felt while eating it, be still and listen to your body. Learn body awareness. Do you feel comfortable, full or over full? Are you bloated now, or maybe even for the rest of the day? Do you feel slightly jittery, or like you want to take a nap? Maybe your mouth is dry. Are you lacking in energy, physically and mentally? Can you focus on anything or concentrate on a task needing to be done?

- Once you are in tune and listening to your body, you will become aware of how you feel after certain foods. The ability to connect back to those feelings when cravings or emotions urge you to step outside of your healthy eating lifestyle helps you to make better choices for your body, and you will find you are less likely to opt for unhealthy foods over the healthy ones. This becomes easier as time goes on, with new healthy habits forming.

- Learn to love colours! *"What does that have to do with food?"* I hear you ask. Take a look at all the foods out there that offer our bodies vitamins and minerals and are highly nutritious. They are vibrant in colour—green, red, purple, white, orange, yellow, and even blue. Then take a look at the foods that aren't so good for us and notice how dull they appear. They also have a low energy vibration whereas fruits and vegetables are bursting with energy.

- Take all of this in when you are out buying your fruit and veg. Stand still for a moment and focus on the colours around you, notice how bright and beautiful they look and feel. When preparing your fruit and veg for eating, take the opportunity at that moment to give thanks and be grateful you have access to this wonderful source of health and energy. Imagine your body being replenished and full of vitamins and minerals from head to toe, while eating these foods.

- Use visions; imagine yourself eating healthy food and your body and soul getting healthier day by day because of it. See yourself healthy (not thin). Envision all the things you want to do once you are at your optimum health. Imagine yourself saying "no" to the foods that aren't beneficial to your health. See yourself walking away from the foods that have no benefit to your health, and watch yourself stride toward the foods that are full of nutrients.

- If you don't like to exercise, then imagine going for strolls in a nice area; by the water if possible, in a nice park or a pretty walking track with trees and flowers. Even just choosing a couple of nice streets close to home is a start. Make sure you actually go for the walk, don't just imagine it. You could ask a friend to join you if you think you will have trouble getting started on your own.

- Envision yourself becoming more active and actually participating in sessions with a personal trainer or going to the gym on a regular basis. Maybe you would prefer a team sport or yoga and pilates. There are a lot of options. Imagine getting active in anything you would like to do, and then find a way to get out there and do it.

- Now it's time to walk the path of a healthy lifestyle, and most of all, enjoy eating, living and breathing a healthy life. See it for what it is—a chance to live life to the fullest, and the ability to get the most out of you, everyday.